Breast cancer has invaded my body,
but it need not invade my spirit.
There may be scars on my chest,
but there need not be scars on my heart.

Judy Kneece

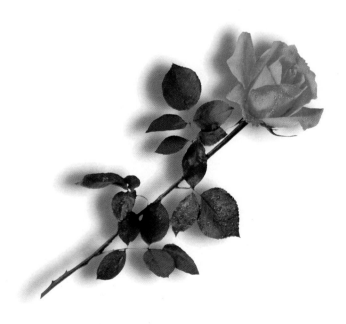

Your Breast Cancer Treatment Handbook

Your guide to understanding the disease,
treatments, emotions and recovery
from breast cancer

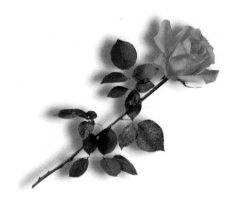

Judy C. Kneece, RN, OCN
Breast Health Specialist

EduCare Publishing
P.O. Box 280305
Columbia, South Carolina 29228

Copyright © 2002 Judy C. Kneece
4th Revised Edition 2001; 3rd Revised Edition 1998; 2nd Revised Edition 1997; 1st Edition 1995.
ISBN 1-886665-10-9
Library of Congress Catalog Card Number: 98-093040
Printed in the United States of America
Published by EduCare Inc.

For orders, contact:

EduCare Publishing
211 Medical Circle
West Columbia, SC 29169
803-796-6100 Voice
803-796-4150 Fax; E-Mail: educare@ix.netcom.com
Internet Site: www.cancerhelp.com

Photographs by Rick Smoak
Illustrations by Debra Strange

Publisher's Cataloging-in-Publication

Kneece, Judy C.
    Your breast cancer treatment handbook : your guide to
      understanding the disease, treatments, emotions and recovery
      from breast cancer / Judy C. Kneece.— 4th ed.
      p. cm. — (EduCare library series)
      Includes bibliographical references and index.
    LCCN: 98-093040
    ISBN: 1-886665-10-9

    1. Breast—Cancer—Patients. 2. Cancer—Treatment.   I. Title. II. Series.

    RC280.B8K54 2001   616.99'44906
                                       QB100-812

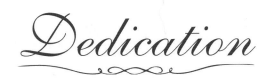

Dedication

This book is dedicated to all of the brave women and their families who have faced the pain and emotional recovery from breast cancer and now serve as my inspiration for this handbook.

My appreciation is extended to the hundreds of patients who shared openly and honestly, as I served as their primary care nurse. Their open expression of their fears, hopes and questions during their breast cancer experience made this book possible. From the privilege of being there with them, I learned the basic educational and recovery needs of women.

To my sister-in-law, Gloria Kneece Stills, who allowed me to share every step of her breast cancer experience physically and emotionally, I owe much of my motivation to learn more and share with other women.

I extend to Cindy Dreher, MPH, MAT, a special debt of gratitude for her support and encouragement throughout this project and her advocacy for breast cancer patients. To those who served as her source of inspiration, I offer a tribute of honor: to her mother, Nell Dreher, breast cancer survivor, and her best friend, Francee Lang Giles, who bravely fought the battle of breast cancer.

My special thanks to Henry Patrick Leis, Jr., MD, FACS, breast surgeon, and his late wife, Winogene Leis, RN, for their encouragement and support in the writing of this workbook and their contributions to women's health.

My gratefulness to Tricia Brown, my editor and editor of *Coping* magazine, for her encouragement for me to make this a book filled with hope as well as facts. Her dedication to this project and compassion for all of the women fighting the battle with breast cancer has been a source of encouragement and strength to me.

A large measure of appreciation is extended to Carolyn Brennan, my executive assistant, for her unfailing support to meet my needs, making it possible for me to revise this book while keeping up with my teaching and speaking schedule, and to Dr. Tom Smith for his expertise and insightful contributions to my writing.

Finally, I dedicate this book to my husband, Bill, and my daughters, Melanie and Sheila, who have supported me every step of my way with their encouragement and support in my mission to educate women about their cancer. Without the personal support and encouragement of Bill, this book would have never become a reality.

Someone once asked, "Have you had breast cancer?" My reply was, "No, my body has not, but my heart has been diagnosed many hundreds of times as I shared the pain my patients were feeling." It is to those of you who now face the same experiences that I make my final dedication. You are the reason for this book!

❧ ❧ ❧

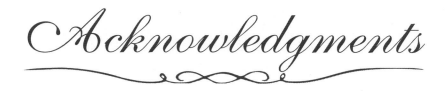

Acknowledgments

Cindy Dreher, MPH, MAT

Tricia Carter Brown, Editor, Layout and Design

Debra Strange, Artist, Illustrator

Dr. Henry Patrick Leis, Jr, Breast Surgeon

Dr. Edward Dalton, Breast Surgeon

Dr. David Krag, Breast Surgical Oncologist

Dr. Richard Fine, Breast Surgical Oncologist

Dr. Kevin Hughes, Breast Surgeon

Dr. Rosemary Lambert-Falls, Medical Oncologist

Dr. Marianna Maldonado, Psychiatrist

Dr. Patsy Lill, Pathology Professor

Dr. Elizabeth Wofford, Pathologist

Dr. Ervin B. Shaw, Pathologist

Dr. Frederick Greene, Breast Surgeon

Jerry Kennedy, MN, RNCS, Clinical Nurse Specialist

Constance A. Roche, MSN, RNCS

Dr. Gabriel de Freitas, Surgical Oncologist, and **Sylvia de Freitas, RN**

Wayne Buff, RPh, and **Nancy Roberts, MS, RPh**, USC College of Pharmacy

Myraid Genetic Laboratories and OncorMed

Debbie Saslow, Ph.D., American Cancer Society

Harriett Barrineau, Breast Cancer Survivor

About the Author

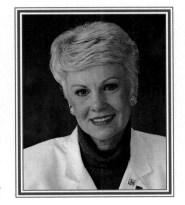

Judy C. Kneece, RN, OCN is a certified oncology nurse with a specialty in breast cancer and a MammaCare® Specialist. She received training at the Mind/Body Medical Institute of Harvard Medical School. Judy presently serves as an international Breast Health Consultant for hospitals and breast health centers in the educational and psychosocial needs of breast cancer patients and their families. She implements a program of comprehensive education, training nurses to fill the breast health education role and setting up a complete program of support for the entire family unit.

Her background as a Breast Health Specialist working in a hospital served as a catalyst for her insights into the needs of women and their families during the breast cancer experience. Judy has personally intervened at the time of diagnosis with hundreds of patients and their families providing emotional support and education about the disease, treatments and recovery. She developed and led support groups for patients and their mates and followed patients throughout the recovery experience.

She is also the author of *Helping Your Mate Face Breast Cancer*, a book for support partners and *Finding A Lump In Your Breast—Where To Go . . . What To Do,* which were both reviewed in the Journal of the National Cancer Institute. Along with *Solving the Mystery of Breast Pain, Solving The Mystery of Breast Discharge* and a computer program featuring over 230 patient education teaching sheets on breast health for clinics, hospitals and physicians' offices. She presently serves as Managed Care Breast Health Editor for *Administrative Radiology* and as a contributing editor for numerous other health magazines. Judy serves on the Board of Trustees and as Secretary for the National Consortium of Breast Centers and acts as Managing Editor for their national newsletter, *The Breast Center Bulletin.* She speaks widely to patients on triumphant survivorship and to the medical community on the topics of comprehensive breast center strategic planning, patient education and support.

Featured on the cover of *Cope, Working in Oncology*, Judy says, "Empowering patients with an understanding of their disease, treatment options and providing tools for recovery management are essential for complete recovery. Breast cancer is more than scars on the breast; it can also scar the heart. We must address the psychological and social issues breast cancer brings if a woman is to master the disease. An understanding of her disease and personal management skills empowers a woman to become an active partner with her health care team and not a passive participant. She must know the advantages and disadvantages of treatment options and the questions she needs to ask about her care. Getting well is more than surgery and treatments; it is a woman understanding the vital role she can play in managing her own recovery."

A Special Note

Harriett Barrineau, Survivor

During my service as a Breast Health Specialist, I had the opportunity to work with Harriett Barrineau. She often wrote to me of her fears, feelings, failures and triumphs during her journey with breast cancer. Her honest and insightful reflections during her diagnosis, treatment and recovery period have become a source of comfort to other women who are just beginning their journeys. Harriett shares with other women what she has experienced. She tells them that they won't always feel hopeful, that there are going to be problems, but that with determination they, too, can make it. She 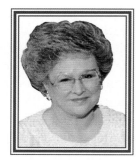 defines survivorship—the quality of using present coping skills and learning new skills to triumph over a seemingly insurmountable task.

Harriett's Story

Harriett was diagnosed with breast cancer in 1990. Because of the characteristics of her tumor, she had a modified radical mastectomy. Surgery was followed by chemotherapy. Over a year later, posture shift, which caused back pain, resulted in Harriett's decision to have a prophylactic second mastectomy and immediate bilateral reconstruction. Today, Harriett works 40 hours a week in her husband's accounting firm and serves as a Reach to Recovery volunteer. Harriett remembers how, after her diagnosis, she searched for people who had already made it through the battle, people who would share with her the ins and outs of the experience. Because she knows the importance of that sharing, she still remains active in a support group.

Her Place in this Book

After completing this manuscript, I realized it contained a great void—the voice of a peer, one who really understands your feelings. As I reviewed my files, I found Harriett's notes to me during her recovery. I asked her permission to include in this book excerpts from her letters. Harriett's quotes in this book serve as the voice of one who knows personally the perils of the journey you are undertaking, a woman who has in fact been where you are and where you are a going—a woman who has survived!

❧ ❧ ❧

Dear Survivor

I almost began this letter "Dear Patient," but then I changed my mind. I do not want you to see yourself or think of yourself as only a patient. You will be a patient for only a short time. You will be a survivor for the rest of your life. I want you to know that you are, from the innermost parts of your being, a breast cancer **survivor**.

Painful as the diagnosis must be, you have joined a host of other women who have experienced the overwhelming anxiety of hearing the words, "You have breast cancer" and are now living examples of survivorship. Among those survivors are:

- Shirley Temple Black
- Jill Eikenberry
- Betty Ford
- Ann Jillian
- Justice Sandra Day O'Connor
- Betty Rollin
- Peggy Fleming
- Carly Simon
- Julia Child
- Linda Ellerbee
- Kate Jackson
- Olivia Newton-John
- Happy Rockefeller
- Diahann Carroll
- Nancy Reagan
- Evelyn Lauder

As you can see from this list, although breast cancer is an unwelcome experience, it is one that can add depth and influence to your life. These well-known women are now advocates in education and support for other women living with cancer. As you begin your journey to understand and recover from breast cancer, be assured that you, too, can master the experience. You can learn, as they learned, how to take the crisis of breast cancer and transform it into an opportunity for personal growth. You can become a triumphant survivor.

As an oncology nurse working only with breast cancer survivors, I have had the privilege to share the intimate experiences of the breast cancer journey with hundreds of women. They shared many of their needs, fears and questions about their disease, treatment and recovery. They also shared many tips which made the experience much easier for them. In this book, I have attempted to share with you the best of what I learned from the patients and physicians with whom I worked.

There is much to know about your disease and recovery. This book is designed to serve as a basic primer for this information. It is not meant to replace or supplant your physicians' instructions. Your physicians and nurses will add additional information and suggest reading materials to help you. Surviving cancer starts with understanding what you can do now that you have cancer. By learning about your disease, you are beginning your journey to survivorship like millions of other women.

Best wishes for a happy and healthy future,

Judy Kneece

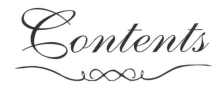

Contents

As Survivors,
we learn that survivorship is an attitude
we adopt. It is the one component of
recovery that no one else can do for us.
We have to decide for ourselves how we
intend to respond to our illness and
how we approach our recovery.
We, alone, decide to become survivors.

Introduction

Your Breast Cancer Treatment Handbook

*"Your entire life will be changed by cancer.
You won't believe it now, but good will come
out of this experience—if you let it."*

~ Harriett Barrineau, survivor

The diagnosis of breast cancer is an unexpected and unplanned event in any woman's life. The emotions become overwhelming as the fears and concerns of surgery and treatment options are discussed and have to be decided upon. There is so much to learn, so much to decide and so little time in which to do it. This handbook is a concise primer of the information that you will need in the following days and months to help you understand your treatment options and how you can best manage.

At the back of this workbook are tear-out worksheets with questions you may want to have answered by your health care team. Women often share that they don't know what to ask when they go for consultations. These sheets will serve as a reference when you visit your physicians as to the type of information you may want to solicit and questions you want answered. Add your own questions to the suggestions.

Acquiring a working knowledge of the language, surgeries and potential treatment options will help restore some sense of control to your life. Your physicians and health care team will be available to answer additional questions and give you information that is specific to your treatment. The more you learn about your breast cancer experience, the better prepared you will be to work as a partner with your health care team in facilitating your physical and emotional recovery. The most important component for a successful recovery is being an educated, determined and optimistic patient. Let's get prepared for recovery!

❧ ❧ ❧

1

"What has happened to us is truly horrible.
But we have a choice.
We can live the rest of our lives
as a memorial service around the event
or we can learn from it
and build an even better life."
~ Gloria Stills

Chapter 1

The Emotional Impact of Breast Cancer

*"My emotions were on a constant roller coaster ride.
One minute I was so grateful I had a good prognosis.
Then anger, fear and depression took over. I realized I was
going to need help working through my emotions."*
~ Harriett Barrineau, survivor

Understanding Your Emotions

Shocked. Scared. Angry. Disappointed. Numb. Irate. Crushed. Disarmed. Furious. Brokenhearted. Speechless. Overwhelmed. These are all terms women have used to describe their emotions upon hearing the words, "You have breast cancer." Most women report that little was heard or remembered after these words were spoken. Their fears took control as they recalled all that they knew in the past about breast cancer. Most often they thought, "Will I die?" Often, they remembered someone who had gone through a similar diagnosis, and, mentally, they substituted themselves into the role. In the midst of this mind-boggling experience, the physician informed them of surgery options and possible treatments. "Overwhelmed" is usually an inadequate word for the experience. How do you begin to work through this complicated maze of decisions and emotions?

Foremost, you must realize that breast cancer is usually a very treatable disease. Survival rates are at an all-time high. Strong emotions are normal for all women at this time. Fears are natural. Most importantly, you need to know that breast cancer is usually not a medical emergency. You can take several weeks without endangering your health to sort through your emotions and to seek answers to your questions. Your physician will discuss this time frame with you. Use this time to gain an understanding of the treatment options you have and the advantages and disadvantages of each. It will be best for you, both emotionally and physically, to take the time to make informed, rational decisions about your treatments.

What Is a Normal Response?

Women experience an array of emotions and respond to the diagnosis according to their basic personalities and previous life experiences. Common to all is that this is a new experience, one that demands a great deal of physical and emotional energy. Most women resort to crying and depression as they sort through their potential losses. Remember, tears are okay. They confirm that you are dealing with reality and are using a very natural and appropriate response to deal with loss. Don't deny yourself the right to grieve. Grieving and tears are signs that your emotional healing has begun.

Some women experience great anger. This anger may be directed against themselves, for not taking steps toward an earlier diagnosis, or toward a physician or even a family member. Anger is an emotion that is used to try to regain control over a situation in which control has been lost. Usually, it serves as a nonproductive way to solve problems; however, it is a natural response. A sense of control will return as you begin to understand and learn about the disease and how you can participate in your recovery. Loss has to be acknowledged before steps to recovery can be effective.

Remember

꙳ Fear, anger, depression and high anxiety are normal emotions at diagnosis. There is no right or wrong way for you to respond emotionally to the diagnosis.

꙳ Breast cancer is not usually a medical emergency. You have time to learn about your diagnosis and treatment options.

Communicating with Family and Friends

Eventually, your thoughts will turn from yourself to your family and friends and the effect this will have on them. They, too, are in pain over your loss. The diagnosis was also a shock to them. Like you, they have a need to express their sad feelings, usually by crying, feeling down and questioning what is ahead as they grieve with you over your loss. This is also a very necessary and natural part of the family's emotional adjustment to your diagnosis.

You can play a very vital part in facilitating their recovery by talking openly of your feelings and allowing them to ask questions and express their thoughts. This is probably one of the hardest parts of the breast cancer experience—open, honest communication. If honest communication begins at the time of diagnosis, it will help both you and your family. Often, we think that if we say nothing or don't let anyone see us crying or feeling depressed, we are making it easier for other people. The opposite is true. Not talking and being dishonest about feelings creates an atmosphere of uncertainty. People don't know what to say or do, and this results in increased anxiety among family members.

Positive attitudes are needed. However, attitudes that seem overly optimistic may also be hard because they set the stage for everyone to be in denial and mask their feelings. The family also needs to see and be able to express the full range of emotions. Begin to share as soon as you can, and ask them to share with you. They may need your permission before they talk because they don't want to "upset" you. Their desire is to help you through this time. When you talk openly, they can find ways that will best help you. Help them to be a part of your recovery by allowing them to do things for you. For example, when they offer to do a chore, accompany you to the doctor or do something special for you, accept the offer. Feeling useful helps their grief and facilitates healing.

Communicating during times of stress may not be easy. You may not find it easy to open up and talk. The one closest to you may not respond if you do open up and share. Breast cancer doesn't change your basic personality or emotional responses to life. If you, your mate or other family members found it difficult to talk before the diagnosis, it may still be difficult to share during this time. However, you need someone to openly share your thoughts and fears in an understanding, nonjudgmental atmosphere. Since you can't force people to participate in communicating, it may be necessary for you to look outside the family unit for someone who can best respond to your needs. Consider your friends, a professional counselor or support group. It is very necessary and helpful for you to locate a support system in which you will be free to communicate and share your feelings.

Studies have shown that women who have good support systems adjust and respond to treatment more effectively. Ask your treating physician or clinic nurses for names of counselors or support groups for breast cancer patients in your area. Breast cancer support groups provide a safe and helpful environment where you can share, learn and receive support from women who know exactly how you feel and what you are facing. The American Cancer Society will also have a list of groups that meet in your area. Find somewhere to communicate your feelings! Acknowledging your emotional responses as normal and communicating openly will set the stage for a successful emotional recovery.

Getting the Facts Straight

Often family and friends who are trying to be helpful will offer you information and suggestions concerning your surgery and treatments. This may only serve to confuse you and increase your anxiety. It is best to listen but not let this interrupt your quest to learn specific information concerning your diagnosis from the professionals guiding your treatment. There have been great advancements in the treatment and management of breast cancer. Drugs have been designed that have changed many of the side effects of chemotherapy. Surgical treatment is often less disfiguring, and survival rates are at an all-time high.

Learning about your disease, surgeries and treatment is important in order to regain a sense of control in your physical recovery. Breast cancer is a disease with many variables. There are approximately 15 types of breast cancer, many that require different surgical management and treatment. For this reason, you cannot compare notes with a friend who had breast cancer, or listen to well-meaning family or friends, because there are too many differences in treatment. Your information needs to come from someone who knows your exact diagnosis and has up-to-date information on the medical management of your disease. Your physician and health care staff will be the best source for this accurate information.

Managing the Breast Cancer Experience

As you are communicating and actively learning about your disease, you will find yourself experiencing mood swings. There will be periods when you feel that you are doing well. Then you may find that you once again feel overwhelmed, questioning "Why?" "What did I do to deserve this?" or saying, "I don't think I can go through this." These are normal responses as you are working through a crisis. You won't always feel in control. Feelings of depression, with periods of crying, may be dispersed throughout your recovery. When these times occur, don't be too hard on yourself for not being "brave." Acknowledge them as normal and then take steps to restore your positive mood by doing whatever seems to help. For some, it helps to get out of the house for a special outing or spending time with friends. You should take steps, whatever helps, to regain a positive mood.

It is also necessary that you monitor your rest during this time. A crisis can drain us of normal energy and require that we get more rest. Listen to your body and get adequate rest. Most women need seven to eight hours of uninterrupted sleep daily. This may mean that you have to ask family members to assume some of your household duties for a time. Plan to include fun events. It is important to do things you enjoy. This will reduce stress as well.

Breast cancer is not an event you would have invited into your life. You will need to learn how to best participate with your health care team in your recovery, but don't allow yourself to make a "career" out of cancer. Try to see it as an experience to rekindle your life. Many women believe that the breast cancer experience caused them to grow into happier and healthier women, adding new dimensions to their lives that they had never taken time to enjoy before. Look at this time as an opportunity to grow, learn and make positive changes in your life. Consider an exercise program. Change your nutritional habits, or take time to start a hobby that brings you joy. A crisis can serve as an opportunity to grow into a physically and emotionally stronger, happier individual. Seek to make this a time of personal growth.

Remember

❧ Tears, anger or depression are all normal initial reactions to your diagnosis.

❧ Identify one or more people to whom you can openly and honestly communicate your fears and concerns. If this person is not in your family unit, reach out to a friend, professional counselor or support group.

❧ Learn about your disease, surgery, treatment and recovery. Information allows you to participate in and understand treatment decisions and restores a sense of control.

❧ Look for opportunities to make this a time of personal growth and take steps to make positive changes in your life.

❧ ❧ ❧

Chapter 2

Your Relationship With Your Mate

*"I needed reassurance from my husband.
I needed to hear, 'I love you.' I needed attention from him.
His faith had to be strong enough for both of us for a short time. But,
later, I realized he also needed support. He, too, was hurting. He found
this unique source of understanding in a mates' support group"*

~ Harriett Barrineau, survivor

At diagnosis, mates are confronted with the same surprise and face the same overwhelming emotions as you. Yet, in the midst of all of this, they often strive to be strong, understanding and supportive. The way mates respond to this crisis will also be determined by their basic personalities and previous coping experiences. Behaviors may vary among people, but under it all are the basic emotions of fear, loss and uncertainty. A mate's love for you causes a strong emotional experience and an extreme feeling of helplessness when you are diagnosed with breast cancer. This is one thing they cannot fix. In an interview concerning support partners, Dr. Marilyn T. Oberst stated:

> *Learning to live with cancer is no easy task. Learning to live with **someone else's** cancer may be **even more difficult,** precisely because **no one** recognizes just how hard it is to **deal** with someone else's cancer.*

Communicating With Your Mate

It is difficult to see you, the one they love, suffering emotionally and physically. Some mates may quietly withdraw emotionally as they sort out the situation mentally. They may not say anything. Others may be very verbal. Remember, this is a new experience for them also. They, too, are hurting emotionally and often feel inadequate in their responses. You can help them by sharing your needs **verbally**. Do not wait, hoping that they will know what you need them to do or how you wish for them to respond. Most mates want to meet their partners' needs and to be helpful, but they are not sure **how** to respond.

7

Recent studies by Dr. Oberst show that during the first six months, some mates may experience greater degrees of emotional problems after a diagnosis than the patient because of their unaddressed fears and the anxiety created by not knowing what is expected of them in their new role as a support partner. You can help by encouraging your mate to talk to others who understand the role of a support partner. Call your cancer treatment center or local American Cancer Society office for the name of support groups for partners or ask for the name of a volunteer. Chaplains working in cancer treatment centers are an excellent source of support because of their understanding of the unique stressors that families face with a cancer diagnosis. Encourage your mate to reach out to others to have their own needs met.

Cancer is a family affair. It emotionally pressures every member of the family. An essential part of healing and recovery is allowing each person to handle the pressures in a way that matches their basic coping skills. When members get stuck emotionally, it is usually because communication is blocked and emotions are not being shared. Cancer presents not only a challenge to family unity between mates, but also an opportunity to strengthen bonds and increase love, respect and understanding.

Changes in the Sexual Relationship

"What effect will my diagnosis and surgery have on my intimate relationship?" "Will I still be loved?" "How will my new body image affect our sexual relationship?" These thoughts are in the back of most women's minds. They are valid questions which need to be explored and understood. Intimate relationships are built on mutual love, trust, attraction, shared interests and common experiences in life. Breast cancer will **not change** these shared feelings.

What may change is how you view your body and how that can affect your sexual intimacy. The physical aspect of lovemaking may temporarily change because of loss of energy resulting from your treatments. However, you can resume your sexual relationship as soon as you feel able. You are still the same loving person your mate selected and loves. You can bring a new dimension to this relationship by openly discussing your feelings about the changes in your body image. Try to communicate honestly about these concerns.

Often, you will need to be the one to initiate the discussion of these fears or needs. Your mate may feel these issues are too personal or sensitive. It is helpful if these concerns are addressed as soon as you are diagnosed. Allowing time to pass only makes the conversations more difficult and walls of silence easier to build.

Early viewing of your incision area is very helpful in restoring the relationship and preventing distance between you and your partner. After surgery, you may feel embarrassed or afraid to talk about your changed body image or to be seen nude by your mate. These feelings are best confronted and faced early. Viewing the incision is a necessary step. It has been proven that, if you share openly, these feelings can be overcome. **Accepting the changes and reaffirming your love and joy of being alive and together will help you work through these feelings.**

Mates often fear that their physical closeness may cause pain or injury to the incision site. It is helpful when you share your need for physical closeness and what is comfortable or uncomfortable to you. Many times what women mistakenly sense as sexual rejection is really an effort on the part of the mate to protect the one they love. Therefore, state your desire for physical contact and share what is pleasurable. This will reduce the unspoken fear in your mate's mind concerning physical intimacy.

Open communication will decrease anxiety for both you and your mate, enabling your personal and sexual relationship to grow even stronger. There may be a period of adjustment, but most couples put their fears behind them and reestablish a satisfying and loving relationship. By sharing both the troubles and triumphs of cancer openly, you and your partner will have the opportunity to strengthen bonds of affection, trust and commitment.

Remember

- Your mate suffers emotionally from the diagnosis, just as you do.

- Most mates are unsure about how best to help.

- Adapting to the role of support person requires open communication. You must let your mate know how to best help during the experience. You must verbalize your needs and express your desires.

- Encourage your mate to reach out for support from others who understand the unique needs of a support partner.

- Intimate relationships are based on love, trust, shared interests and common experiences; breast cancer does not change this.

- Sexual intimacy after surgery is dependent upon open communication. Discuss your change in body image, view the incision early and verbalize your need for continued intimacy.

- Breast cancer can bring a couple closer and strengthen the bonds of affection, trust and commitment.

Support Partner's Guide Available
A companion to this book is available for your support partner, *Helping Your Mate Face Breast Cancer*. This book is designed as a guide to help a mate understand how to best help you while understanding their own emotional responses to the diagnosis. It addresses the unique emotional issues that a mate faces during a partner's breast cancer diagnosis and explains what they can do. Ask your health care provider about this book or you may order it from the form provided in the back of this book.

As Survivors,
we take a misfortune of life
and change it into something that
produces personal growth and
somehow benefits others.

Chapter 3

How You Can Help Your Children

*"Having always been the caretaker in my
family, I found it difficult to let my four sons know
I needed anything. I finally told them that I needed to talk
about my fears and feelings, even though talking about
Mom's breasts was not the most comfortable subject. Our
love for one another and deep faith in God brought us
closer together during this crisis."*

~ Harriett Barrineau, survivor

Children react to a parent's illness in various ways, according to their ages, developmental stages and personalities. As a parent, you want this illness to create as little negative effect as possible on their lives. How do you handle this situation so that it causes the least amount of emotional distress for the children? From the beginning, tell the truth and answer their questions honestly. Often, it may appear that keeping the facts from them would be more helpful, but this is not wise. Children are very perceptive; they instinctively sense when something is wrong in the family. Not knowing **what** is wrong often will cause them to imagine things, which results in more anxiety than knowing the truth. It is also important that they hear it first from you or the family, not from strangers. When information is presented truthfully, on their level of understanding, they can interact with you and receive answers to their questions and fears. It may be helpful to ask your medical team if they have information on how to talk with children about cancer.

How to Tell Your Children

It is best if you can relay the information yourself. However, you may wish to have your mate or a family member present to help answer questions. Tell your child in non-medical language what is going to happen to you during surgery and treatment. Assure your children

11

you will continue to keep them informed. Take care not to overload them with any more information than is necessary. Encourage them to ask questions. Assure them that it is okay for them or you to feel sad and cry. If you should cry during this time, consider this as normal.

Some children may express anger. Some may be frightened. Some will feel that something they did or did not do caused the disease. However, most children listen and accept what you say with little interruption in their daily routine. As Dr. Pertz, explains in his book, **How Do We Tell The Children?**

> *A child's first question about illness and death is an attempt to gain mastery over frightening images of abandonment, separation, loneliness, pain, and bodily damage. If we err on the side of **overprotecting** them from emotional pain and grief with 'kind **lies**,' we risk **weakening** their coping capacities.* [emphasis added]

Including the Family

One way to use your diagnosis as a time for growth is to allow your children to participate in your illness. Allow them to assume some small household chores according to their ages. Helping around the house will cause them to feel a part of the family unit, fostering a sense of contribution to the good of the family.

Small children often enjoy the slower pace that surgery or treatments bring to their mother. They find the time mother spends lounging around is a special treat. One family had camp-outs in the family room on the weekends their mother had her chemotherapy. Rented movies, prepared-ahead food and sleeping bags beside mom on the sofa became a special event each month. Planning to incorporate the children into the experience removes some of the fears they may have.

Teenagers also have fears, and you need to be honest with them. Keeping them informed is essential. They also need to participate in family chores. Avoid the tendency to overload teenagers—requiring them to give up too much of their social lives. Select ways in which they can help and yet still maintain their independence. Since it may be too overwhelming for your teenager to become your **only** source of open communication, develop several sources of personal support and communication.

The breast cancer experience does **not** have to be a negative experience for the children and teens in your family. It can serve as a time when families grow stronger. However, if your child should experience difficulty in adjusting, contact your clinic or physician for the name of a counselor in this area. Written material is available from the American Cancer Society on the topic of how to help children cope with a parent's illness.

Remember

- Children need to be told the truth, at the level of their understanding, by you or a close family member.

- They need their questions answered honestly.

- Truthfulness, coupled with love, will enable your child to grow stronger through this family crisis.

- Children need to feel a part of the family by assisting with household chores.

- Teens need to maintain their social life as much as possible and not become the only source of communication or support for the parent.

- Breast cancer does not have to be a negative experience for children. It can serve as a time when families grow stronger.

*As Survivors,
we choose hope after loss.
We choose to look at what we can do now
that tragedy has invaded our lives.
We acknowledge our loss and nurse our pain,
but we move on to make the tragedy a source of
motivation for a new direction in our lives.*

Chapter 4

Calming Your Fears

*"My husband's first reaction to my diagnosis was
that we had been given a death sentence.
Mine was just the opposite. I saw death as the easy choice.
My greatest fear was having to live
with the aftermath of breast cancer."*

~ Harriett Barrineau, survivor

Fear is a paralyzing force. As a nurse working with breast cancer patients, I have listened to the many fears that diagnosis brings. Often the fears become overwhelming as they are mentally sorted through. In our support group, women were often surprised to hear other women express the same fears. Yes, fears are common to all. However, they may vary in degree of intensity according to your personality, previous coping experiences and your present support system. The most commonly expressed fears are:

- Will I die? How do I need to plan for the future?
- Will I live to see my children grow up?
- Are they telling me the truth?
- How can I protect my loved ones from the pain this causes?
- Can I cope after I have my breast removed?
- Will treatment be painful? Will treatment work?
- Can I deal with the side effects of treatment?
- Will I become a burden to my family?
- What will this cost, and can we afford it?
- Will I still be sexually attractive? Can I still be physically attractive?
- How will this affect my job?

◆ How will I know if cancer recurs?

◆ **I feel helpless. What can I do about cancer?**

How do you handle your fears? First, know that fear is natural. In fact, women who do not express fear are those who are most at risk psychologically. Disarming fear begins with recognizing its presence, expressing the fear to the appropriate person and taking steps of action against the fear. Do not hold on to your fears in silence. Express them. Often, when a fearful emotion is brought out in the open, it begins to lose some of its intensity. When it is expressed, strategies can be developed to deal with the fear. Expressing fear can start with your own search for the fears which are plaguing you the most at this time.

Make a list of the fears that are clouding your mind (see the example below). Be honest. You do not have to show anyone the list. After you have made your list, in a column beside the fear, list who the fear involves. If another person is involved, such as your mate or physician, express your fear to them. Think about the fear and actions that you can take to understand or to change the fear.

Fear	Person(s) Involved	Things I Can Do
"Will I still be sexually attractive?"	Mate	Express fear. Purchase attractive lingerie. Express desire for closeness. Plan special times.
"Are they telling me the truth?"	Physician Nurses	Ask for honesty and all the facts. Read about my disease.
"What can I do about cancer?"	Support Group Professional Counselor	Attend a support group. Ask for the name of a counselor.

A worksheet for listing your fears and your planned strategies to disarm them (similar to the one above) is located on page 159 in the reference section of this book. Begin by listing your fears. When you are ready to express your fears to the appropriate person, state your fear questions using "**I**" language. Example: "**I** am very concerned about the effect of my surgery on our sexual relationship. **I** don't want it to change." You may say to your physician, "**I** want to know all of the details about my disease and the side effects of treatment."

Fear can be a great impediment to recovery. Expressing the fear, determining your resources and developing a plan of action will cause the fear to be less of a threat. Communicate openly with your health care team and your support partners. Verbalizing the fears allows them to help you seek a strategy to deal with the fear. All uncertainty will never be alleviated, but the fears can certainly be brought to a manageable level.

Sources which have been proven to assist in the management of fear are support groups, professional counselors and spiritual faith. From these sources a wealth of strength may be gained to deal with the diagnosis of cancer. As your physician and health care team are working to eradicate the cancer from your body, you can work to provide an emotional environment in your body as free from stress and fear as possible.

Support Groups

Support groups are a "safe" place to express your fears and have your cancer questions answered by those who truly understand. You may have loving support from your family and friends, but often they do not seem quite able to understand what you really feel. In a breast cancer support group, the shared experiences of other women serve to restore the adaptive process needed to resume your fighting spirit. It is helpful to see those who are months ahead of you living full, productive lives after mastering the crisis of breast cancer. They have many tips and much encouragement to share with you. Avail yourself of this source of strength and understanding.

Ask your treatment team for names of groups or call your local American Cancer Society. The National Alliance of Breast Cancer Organizations has a national list of breast cancer support groups. One may be in your area (the number is in the reference section). When you have identified a support group or groups, you may wish to call and ask about the organization and goals of the group. Select a group which is affiliated with a medical facility, if possible. These groups are usually facilitated by professionals who have an understanding of breast cancer and are able to get accurate answers to your questions.

Visit the group at least twice before making a judgment. If you do not feel you had your needs met, visit another group if possible. Try to avoid any group that is allowed to become a "pity party" and select one which offers education and sharing among participants and promotes an optimistic approach to recovery.

It is also helpful if your mate can attend a support group. Often, mates have very few people with whom they can confide and receive helpful support. Ask about local support groups for your mate. A companion to this book for support partners, *Helping Your Mate Face Breast Cancer,* is available as a support guide from EduCare Publishing, offering tips on how mates can aid in their role as supporters.

Some cancer centers also offer educational classes for younger children. This allows them to meet with other children and learn about cancer and cancer treatment on their level of understanding. Ask about children's classes for educational support.

Over 90 percent of patients feel that support groups were helpful to their recovery. Women who participate in groups or seek support from professionals have been proven to adjust more quickly both physically and emotionally than non-participants. Support groups are a way to reduce your fears and get answers to your questions.

Professional Counseling

Support groups are a valuable source of free information and support. However, some women do not feel comfortable in a large group or do not have access to a support group because of time or distance. If you find that a support group cannot meet your needs, ask your health care team for the name of a specialized counselor, therapist or psychiatrist. This is not a sign of weakness but of strength. Seeking appropriate support is as necessary as seeking appropriate medical treatment. The difference is you may have to express your need for this service.

Individual counseling allows you to express your feelings and fears in an atmosphere of trust and support. Your selected counselor helps you plan strategies to make this crisis a manageable event in your life. This is usually short-term crisis counseling.

Spiritual Faith

Inherent in each of us is a deep need for understanding our existence and our future. Cancer causes a real threat to the sense of safety and forces these issues to be foremost in the mind. Struggling to understand "why," "how" and "what about tomorrow" is found in one's faith. It will be helpful if you reach out and seek the help of your spiritual counselor during this time. If you do not have a pastor, priest or spiritual leader, ask your hospital for the name of the chaplaincy service. Chaplains are trained in dealing with the adjustment to the crisis of cancer. Avail yourself of this service.

In the book *Cancervive* Susan Nessim shares her feelings as a cancer survivor:

> *"Cancer has taken us on an amazing journey. When we look in the mirror we may see our faces as unchanged, but the person they belong to has undergone a **spiritual metamorphosis**. We have shed our old skins. Now we must assess who we've become and where we're headed. . . . We've gained new insights into the depths of our spiritual strength, physical resiliency and courage." [emphasis added]*

Looking at the cancer experience through the eyes of spiritual faith gives the experience meaning and purpose. Susan continues,

> *"In the school of life, cancer survivors feel as if they've just completed an accelerated course—not that anyone, given the choice, would sign up for that course again. But for those fortunate enough to have gained a new perspective, the lessons learned are as precious as life itself."*

18

Remember

- 🙖 Fear is common to **all** women diagnosed with breast cancer. You are not unusual because of your fears. Relax, you are normal.

- 🙖 Fear is not a sign of weakness.

- 🙖 Keep in mind, fears vary in intensity according to an individual's personality, previous coping experiences and support systems.

- 🙖 Fears lose their power when expressed openly and when steps are taken to disarm them.

- 🙖 The first step is to name the fear questions which cloud your mind. Write them down.

- 🙖 Support groups offer much emotional help and answer many fear questions.

- 🙖 Some women are not comfortable in a large group and can benefit greatly from individual professional counseling.

- 🙖 Spiritual faith is a very strong component in giving meaning to fear and providing a sense of strength to surmount the crisis of diagnosis. Reach out for spiritual understanding.

"Fear is conquered by action.
When we challenge our fears, we defeat them.
When we grapple with our difficulties, they lose their hold upon us.
When we dare to face the things which scare us, we open the door to freedom."
~ Wynn Adams

🙖 🙖 🙖

Refer to the tear-out worksheet, "Managing My Fears," located at the back of the book.

*As Survivors,
we fight back at adversity with a
desire to grow and learn.
We find resources to give us the
skill to handle what life has brought
our way. We put priority on
learning about our adversity rather
than fleeing in panic. We read,
listen and reach out to those who can
give us understanding.*

Chapter 5

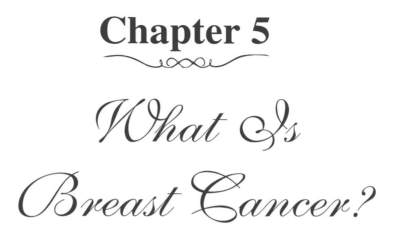

What Is Breast Cancer?

"Breast cancer is not the
unconquerable enemy I thought it was."
~ Harriett Barrineau, survivor

Breast cancer is not a sudden occurrence, but a process which has been developing for a period of time. Therefore, when a biopsy confirms a cancerous breast tumor, you are not facing a medical emergency. You have time to get answers to your questions and learn about your particular disease and treatment options. Most physicians recommend surgery within several weeks of biopsy. There are exceptions; for example, cancer in the lymphatic system (also known as Inflammatory Carcinoma) requires immediate treatment with chemotherapy for maximum control. Ask your physician what recommendations will be made regarding your particular tumor. Tests performed on your tumor will reveal cell type and estimate whether the tumor is a very slow growing or a more rapidly growing tumor.

Some tumors will characteristically spread more rapidly to other parts of the body, while others do not seem to spread as readily. Breast cancer spreads to other parts of the body through the lymphatic system or the blood system. The spread of the cancer can be local (in the area of the breast), regional (in the nodes or area near the breast) or distant (to other organs of the body).

What Causes Breast Cancer?

The female breast is a very complicated glandular organ and is the site of the most common cancer in women–breast cancer. No one knows exactly what causes breast cancer. Genetics, having a family history of breast cancer, increase the risk. Other identified possible causes have been environmental carcinogens, viruses, radiation therapy and life-style factors, including diet and hormonal function.

Cancer begins when the cells of the breast undergo changes. The normal cell converts into a cell which has an uncontrolled growth pattern. The cancer cells continue to divide and grow and may spread to other parts of the breast and then to other parts of the body if not removed. The cancer cells can invade neighboring tissues and spread throughout the body, establishing new growths at distant sites. This process is called **metastasis.**

Types of Breast Cancer

Approximately 15 different types of breast cancer have been identified. The term **carcinoma** is used by physicians to describe a malignant or cancerous growth. Tumors which develop from different types of breast tissue, in different parts of the breast, may have varying characteristics of development.

Breast cancers are named according to the part of the breast in which they develop. Cancers beginning in the ducts are called **ductal carcinomas** and comprise the largest number of cancers occurring in women. Cancers beginning in the lobules are called **lobular carcinomas** and account for a small percentage of diagnoses. If the cancer grows through the cell walls it is called an **infiltrating** or **invasive** carcinoma. **In situ** carcinomas are cancers which are still contained within the walls of the breast area in which they developed. They have not invaded surrounding tissue.

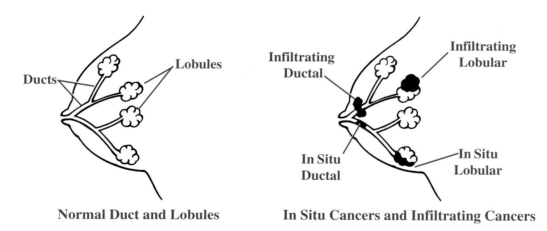

Normal Duct and Lobules   **In Situ Cancers and Infiltrating Cancers**

Most breast cancers occur in the upper, outer part of the breast, near or in the area from the nipple back toward the underarm area (axillary tail). Interestingly enough, more cancers occur in the left breast than the right breast.

Some breast cancers grow rapidly, while others are very slow-growing. Breast cancers have been shown to double in size every 23 to 209 days. A tumor which doubles every 100 days (the estimated average doubling time) would have been in your body approximately eight to ten years when it reaches one centimeter in size (3/8 inch)—the size of the tip of your smallest finger. The cancer begins with one damaged cell and doubles until it is detected on mammography or by finding a lump. The cancer must be surgically removed from the body, killed with chemotherapy or radiation therapy or controlled with hormonal therapy. Some people believe that cancers may grow in spurts and the doubling time may vary at different times. However, by the time a one centimeter tumor is found, the tumor has already grown from one cell to approximately 100 billion cells.

The Role of the Lymphatic System

Lymph nodes play an important role in the discussion of your treatment decisions. It is helpful if you understand how the lymphatic system affects many decisions. The lymphatic system serves as the sewage system for cellular waste in the body. The lymph vessels follow closely beside the blood vessels and receive the cell's waste products. This waste is carried by the vessels and filtered through rounded areas of the lymph system, referred to as the **lymph nodes**. Nodes appear as small round capsules and vary from pinhead to olive-size. Lymphocytes and monocytes (components of fluid which fight infection) are produced in the nodes, and the nodes act as filters to stop bacteria, cellular waste and cancer cells from entering the blood stream. Lymph nodes may also serve as metastatic sites—places where cancer has spread from the original site to nodes, now referred to as **secondary sites**.

Three percent of the lymphatic fluid leaving the breast is drained in the lymph nodes located in the area of the breast bone, called **internal mammary nodes**. Ninety-seven percent of the fluid is drained through the nodes located in the area of the arm pit, referred to as the **axillary nodes**. There are three levels of nodes in the axillary area. Your surgeon may remove several nodes from one or several levels, a procedure called **axillary sampling** or **axillary dissection** when all the nodes under the arm are removed. The number of nodes in each level varies from person to person.

Nodes are removed to determine whether your cancer has moved from the breast into the node area. The term **negative nodes** means that your lymph nodes did not have any evidence of cancer. **Positive nodes** indicate that the cancer was found in the lymph nodes. Your surgeon will tell you how many nodes were removed during your surgery and how many were found to have cancer cells present. Treatment decisions are often based on the number of nodes in which cancer cells are found. Two important factors that determine your oncologist's treatment plan are the **number** of **positive nodes** and the **size** of your **tumor.**

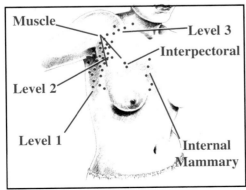 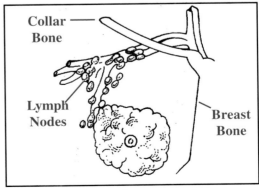

Axillary Lymph Nodes—One or three levels may be removed.
Level 2 nodes are behind the pectoralis minor muscle.

Sentinel Lymph Node Surgery

Sentinel lymph node surgery is a **new** procedure that identifies the first nodes (sentinel) that receive lymphatic fluid from a cancerous tumor, thus identifying the lymphatic drainage pattern. Tumors may drain to different node chains in the breast, according to the position of the tumor. This procedure identifies the chain and the nodes most likely to show if cancer has metastasized from the original tumor to the regional lymph node area. (Refer to previous page for illustration of lymph node drainage patterns in the breast.) This identification allows the surgeon and the pathologist to have a reliable guide for more accurate node evaluation.

Sentinel lymph node surgery is now under study in clinical trials and may not be available in all surgical centers. Ask your health care team if this procedure is available in your facility.

If available, the procedure is performed as part of the surgical removal of the tumor. The area surrounding the tumor is injected with a dye and/or radiographic substance several hours before surgery. Before the incision is made on the breast, a hand-held gamma-detection probe identifies for the surgeon the area of greatest intake of the injected radiographic material. This guides the surgeon to the lymphatic chain that drains the tumor, allowing removal of the nodes stained by the dye, the sentinel nodes. This process also identifies for the pathologist the nodes most likely to have cancerous cells present.

Correctly identifying the draining nodes can significantly improve the accuracy of selecting the nodes to remove surgically and evaluate for spread of the cancer. It may also prevent unnecessary removal of nodes which may not be in the lymphatic drainage field of the tumor. Reducing the number of nodes removed during surgery can reduce the potential for lymphedema, a swelling from lymphatic fluid accumulation in the arm. Lymphedema can cause discomfort in the arm, depression from having to deal with the body image change, and increase the likelihood of an infection in the arm if any type of injury should occur.

Summary:

Surgery and treatment with chemotherapy, radiation therapy or hormonal therapy can all vary because of the differences in types of cancer, the size of the tumor, potential lymph node involvement or documented metastasis, aggressiveness of the tumor and hormonal sensitivity. Therefore, it is necessary for you to communicate with health care professionals who have access to your particular disease type when seeking any specific information or advice on your breast cancer treatment.

Remember

- Breast cancer is not a sudden occurrence; it has been developing for years.

- Breast cancer is usually **not** a medical emergency. You usually have time to gather information and get answers to your questions before surgery and treatments.

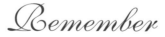

Chapter 6

Surgical Treatment Decisions

*"I was frightened by how fast things were happening.
I felt totally ignorant about breast cancer
and had no idea where to turn
for information or education."*

~ Harriett Barrineau, survivor

When your acute emotional stress is diminished, you may have many concerns about your diagnosis which need to be clarified. Many women say they were not prepared to hear the diagnosis and that everything the doctor said after the word "cancer" was hazy in their minds. You may want to list your questions and call the physician's office to schedule an appointment to receive accurate answers. Make this list with the person who accompanied you to the initial appointment. Before your visit, it will be helpful to begin to read and acquire a basic understanding of the medical terms used and some of the treatment options that may be offered. This booklet contains that basic information. Your physician can recommend other books or brochures that will be helpful.

Today, women have the opportunity to participate and decide, with their physicians, which type of treatment will meet their personal needs and give the best chance for disease-free survival. It is important for you to understand why you are, or are not, offered certain treatment modalities. As an informed patient, you can become an active partner with your physician, understanding the treatments being discussed. It is also helpful if you can select one support person to accompany you to your appointments and participate in this process. This person will be a shoulder you can lean on and can help you remember and evaluate the information that is presented.

Obtaining accurate information about your particular disease is very important. Ask your physician for recommended reading material. Much information is written in women's magazines that is interesting; but often it may not apply to the type of cancer you have and may confuse you. Medical terms sometimes have unusual meanings. Using a glossary to clarify the definitions of words will be helpful. As you read and learn, a sense of understanding will replace much of your fear about breast cancer. (Listed at the end of this book are sources of free medical information that offer up-to-date material on breast cancer. Also listed are suggested reading materials and resource lists to assist you in other areas, in addition to a glossary of breast cancer terms.)

Surgical Treatment Decisions

Surgery is the first line of defense against most breast cancers. Your surgeon will discuss with you the best surgery for your diagnosis. Your surgeon will consider the following facts in determining which surgery best suits your needs:

- Type of tumor—The type was diagnosed by biopsy and confirmed by the pathology report. There are approximately 15 cell types of breast cancer that vary in tumor growth rate (how aggressively the tumor may spread to other organs and its potential for occurring in the other breast).

- Size of the tumor—Sizes are given in centimeters (cm) and millimeters (mm). (10 mm equal 1 cm; 1 cm equals 3/8 inch; one inch equals 2.5 cm)

- Size of your breast—Some breasts may be too small in comparison to the size of the lump to give good cosmetic appearance when the lump is removed.

- Location in your breast—Tumors under the nipple sometimes will not give a suitable cosmetic look when the lump is removed.

- Possible tumor involvement in lymph nodes.

- Appearance of mammogram—Determines if your tumor may be multicentric (occurring in more than one place in the breast). This is sometimes evidenced by microcalcifications (small calcium deposits) or mammographic abnormalities.

- Involvement of other structures (skin, muscle, chest wall, bone or other organs).

- Your desire for reconstruction now or later and the desired outcome for the reconstructive surgery (breast enlargement, reduction or matching present size).

- Your general health and any treatment limitations due to your present health.

- Which surgery will give you the best chance for a cure.

- Which surgery will give you the best cosmetic results.

- Which surgery will give you the best functional results for your arm and shoulder.

- Which surgery is associated with the fewest short-term and long-term complications.

- What your priorities are regarding the surgery.

Each tumor must be evaluated in terms of its unique and specific features and what surgery will be best for you. Some types of breast cancer may require chemotherapy treatments before surgery. Discuss the above considerations with your surgeon and ask any questions which will help you both make the decision best suited to your needs.

Types of Surgery

Surgery for breast cancer includes several types of surgical procedures. Some types remove the breast (**mastectomy**), and others remove the tumor and varying degrees of the remaining breast tissue (**lumpectomy**). These common terms may describe various amounts of tissue removal, and you will need to clarify with your surgeon which of the exact procedures will be used. Listed below are the basic types of surgical procedures and descriptions of the tissues, usually removed. After each description, one drawing illustrates the amount of tissue removed, and another drawing illustrates how your body will appear after the surgery. Surgical incisions can vary with different surgeons. A blank illustration (page 163) is provided at the back of this book for your surgeon to draw the procedure which will be used for your surgical treatment and how your scar should appear afterwards.

Breast Conservation Surgery (Lumpectomy)

Surgery that conserves your breast is commonly referred to as a "lumpectomy." Breast conservation surgery preserves your body image because it saves the majority of the breast tissue, including the nipple and the areola. However, there are some reasons that breast conserving surgery may not be the best surgical option.

Factors That May Disqualify You for Breast Conserving Surgery

◆ Pregnancy (if radiation therapy will be required after surgery)

◆ More than one primary tumor in the breast

◆ Mammogram with evidence of suspicious scattered microcalcifications

◆ Location of the tumor in the breast (in cases where there may be poor cosmetic results—example, when the tumor is located under the nipple)

◆ Size of tumor (if the tumor is too large or the breast is too small in relation to the size of the tumor, then there will be poor cosmetic results)

◆ Prior radiation therapy to breast or chest area

◆ Collagen vascular disease (lupus, scleroderma, etc.)

◆ Severe chronic lung disease (because you may not be a candidate for radiation therapy)

◆ Very large pendulous breast (indicates you may not be a good candidate for radiation therapy)

◆ Evidence of remaining cancer in ducts surrounding tumor (indicating there may be a high risk for recurrence)

◆ Restrictions on travel or transportation to clinic for daily radiation for five to six weeks

There are several types of breast conserving surgeries. Different amounts of tissue may be removed according to the size and cell type of your tumor. These variations in the amount of tissue removed have different names. Lymph node removal during breast conserving surgery also varies. Ask your surgeon which of the procedures will be performed and the extent of tissue and lymph node removal you will need to have. There is a separate page (page 163) that your surgeon may fill in for you as to where and how your incision will look after your surgery. The different breast conserving surgeries are defined below:

1. Partial or Segmental Mastectomy

The tumor, overlying skin and an area of tissue around the tumor are removed in this surgery. A portion of the lining of the chest muscle under the tumor and some of the skin may also be removed. Lymph nodes may or may not be removed from a separate incision, approximately two inches in length, under the arm.

2. Tylectomy

The tumor and a wide area of tissue around the tumor are removed during surgery. Lymph nodes may or may not be removed by a second incision under the arm.

3. Lumpectomy

Lumpectomy removes the tumor and a small wedge of surrounding tissue. Lymph nodes may or may not be removed by a separate incision under your arm.

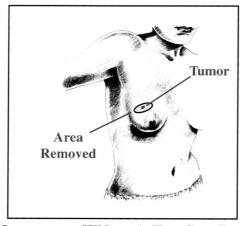

Lumpectomy Without Axillary Sampling

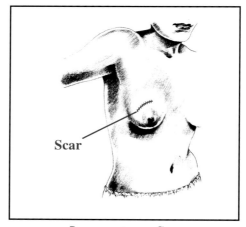

Lumpectomy Scar

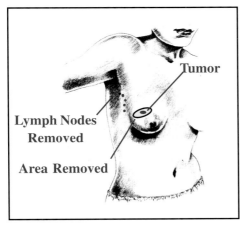

Lumpectomy With Axillary Sampling

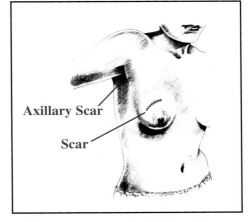

Lumpectomy and Axillary Scars

Incisions for breast conserving procedures appear very similar in relation to the cosmetic appearance of the breast, differing only in accordance to the amount of tissue removed.

Mastectomy

There are several types of mastectomies. Ask your surgeon which of the procedures will be performed and the extent of tissue and lymph node removal you will need to have. There is a separate page (page 163) in the back of this workbook that your surgeon may fill in for you, outlining where and how your incision will look after surgery. The different mastectomies are defined below:

Halsted Radical Mastectomy

This surgery is rarely used today. The Halsted Radical was the most common breast surgery used for over 70 years. It removes the breast, nipple, areola, all underarm lymph nodes and both chest muscles. Because of the removal of the muscles, the chest was left with a cave-type appearance. Medical advances have replaced this procedure with surgeries that are less disfiguring. Because of the rarity of this surgery, it is not pictured.

Modified Radical Mastectomy (Conservative or Limited)

A modified radical mastectomy removes the breast, nipple, areola, underarm lymph nodes and the lining over the chest wall muscles. You may hear the procedure referred to as a "total mastectomy with axillary dissection" which means that the entire breast and some or all of level one and two lymph nodes are removed. The chest muscles and pectoral nerves are not removed.

Full or Complete Modified Radical Mastectomy

A full modified radical mastectomy removes the breast, nipple, areola, all three levels of lymph nodes, small chest muscle, the pectoralis minor, medial pectoral nerve and the lining over the chest wall muscles.

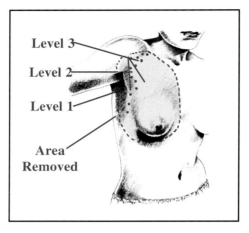

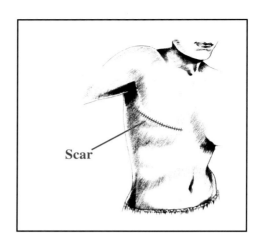

| Mastectomy | Mastectomy Scar |

Total, Simple or Prophylactic Mastectomy

This procedure removes the breast tissue, nipple, areola and possibly some of the underarm lymph nodes that are closest to the breast.

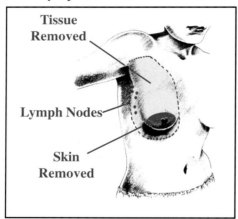

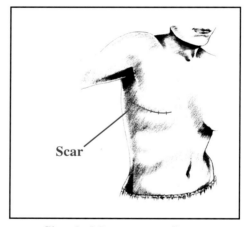

| Simple Mastectomy | Simple Mastectomy Scar |

Skin-Sparing Mastectomy

Skin-sparing mastectomy is a new procedure used when performing a simple or total mastectomy. The method removes the breast tissues from a circular incision around the areola (dark colored circle). The nipple, areola, breast tissues, nodes located near the breast tissues and additional lymph nodes are removed according to the discretion of the surgeon. The procedure is often selected when reconstructive surgery is performed. The sparing of the skin allows reconstructive surgery to be performed with little need for a period of stretching of the skin. Sensitivity of the skin over the reconstructed breast remains intact. The reconstructive incision is made using the normal curve of the breast. This incision is not as visible because it is hidden under the fold of the breast and is concealed by the bra. The incision used to remove the breast is concealed by the reconstruction of a nipple and areola.

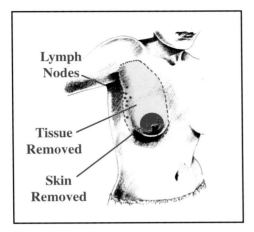

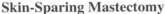

Skin-Sparing Mastectomy

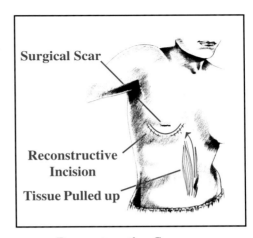

Reconstructive Surgery

Lumpectomy Versus Mastectomy

If your breast and tumor are within certain size limits, your surgeon may offer you the option of a lumpectomy (breast conservation) versus a mastectomy. If you are in the category that gives you the option to choose between a lumpectomy and a mastectomy, the decision may be difficult. This needs to be a decision you make in consultation with your physician, after careful review of the advantages and disadvantages of both. Remember, the option to choose is not available for some types of cancer. **It is imperative that you feel comfortable with the decision.** Studies document that a lumpectomy, even if there is local recurrence, **does not affect survival rate.** However, the inconvenience may come from the necessity to have a second surgery. **Ask your surgeon if there are any additional variables in your surgical decision that may be added to this list.**

Advantages of Lumpectomy

- ◆ Saves a large portion of the breast, usually the nipple and areola
- ◆ Preserves body image
- ◆ You are able to wear your own bras
- ◆ Rarely requires reconstruction or the wearing of a prosthesis
- ◆ Recovery time from surgery is shorter, usually several weeks
- ◆ Slightly shorter hospitalization time or may be performed as outpatient surgery
- ◆ May be psychologically easier to accept, unless the fear of monitoring remaining breast tissue for recurrence is too frightening

Disadvantages of Lumpectomy
- Risk of recurrence of cancer in remaining breast tissue
- Several weeks, usually five to six, of radiation therapy to the remaining breast tissue
- Changes in texture (lumpiness), color (suntanned appearance) and decreased sensation of feeling to the breast after radiation therapy
- Decrease in size of the remaining breast tissues after swelling decreases following radiation treatments
- Monthly breast self-exam on remaining breast tissue (to monitor for recurrence) becomes more difficult because of increased nodularity (lumpiness) from radiation therapy
- Possibility of future second lumpectomy or mastectomy if there is a recurrence

Advantages of Mastectomy
- Removes approximately 95 percent of all the breast gland, including the nipple and areola, thus reducing local recurrence to the lowest degree
- Reconstruction of breast is available using your own body tissue or using synthetic implants

Disadvantages of Mastectomy
- Body image is changed because of the removal of a breast
- Need for prosthesis or reconstruction to restore body image
- Recovery time is slightly longer than for lumpectomy patients, usually several weeks

If you are having problems making your decision, you may wish to speak with a patient who has already made the choice and had one of the procedures. Ask your physician if there is someone who will be willing to talk to you. Your local American Cancer Society's **Reach to Recovery** program coordinator can provide you with a volunteer's name who will be willing to share her lumpectomy/mastectomy experience.

If you are considering a lumpectomy, you may wish to have a consultation with a radiation oncologist to discuss radiation treatments. Often this consultation will give you additional insight that may help you make a more informed decision. (See Chapter 9 for more information on radiation therapy.)

Prophylactic Mastectomy

For some women there may be an option for a prophylactic mastectomy (simple mastectomy) of a breast. A prophylactic mastectomy takes place before cancer has been found. Some women with extremely high risk of breast cancer or precancerous conditions in the breast choose to have this procedure. This elective surgery is a decision made collaboratively between the patient, surgeon and oncologist. A second opinion may be required to ensure that this is a physically and psychologically sound decision. Reasons for which this procedure may be considered include:

- Family history of breast cancer, including first degree relatives who died of the disease
- Repeated breast biopsies for suspicious findings
- Mammograms that show findings that are increasingly difficult to interpret
- Diagnosis of a cancer type that has a high rate of occurrence in both breasts
- When the weight of a very large remaining breast (after mastectomy) creates imbalance, posture changes and back pain
- Overwhelming psychological fear of occurrence in remaining breast
- Desire for bilateral reconstruction with an increase or decrease in the reconstructed breast size

Second Opinions

When a medical diagnosis is serious and the suggested therapy hard to accept, some women feel the need for additional information or a second opinion. Surgery, chemotherapy and radiation therapy deserve serious consideration, and you need all of the information necessary to make an informed decision. A second opinion is obtained from another physician, practicing in the same area of medicine, who reviews your records and offers treatment advice. This opinion may help you feel sure about your treatment decision. **However, for some women, a second opinion may cause anxiety and increase confusion.**

Some insurance providers require second opinions before treatment. You will need to check with your insurance provider on this point. Physicians may refer patients for second opinions in order to validate treatment decisions. It is necessary for you to evaluate your needs and decide if a second opinion would be of assistance to you.

Reasons You May Need a Second Opinion

- If you feel insecure or unsure about what you have been told about surgery or treatments
- If your insurance provider requires a second opinion

◆ If there has been a disagreement or confusion within your family or with your support partner about the right course of action

◆ If you want information about newer therapies not offered by your treatment team

How to Find a Second Opinion

If you feel a second opinion would help you resolve your indecisiveness, ask your treatment team for the names of several physicians qualified in this area. Ask the treatment team to list the pros and cons of each one in order to help you determine who will best suit your needs. You may also call a major cancer treatment center for a referral. Some of the national cancer organizations listed in the reference section of this book will give you the names of the major cancer treatment centers located in your area and the services they provide.

Second opinions are sometimes received through multidisciplinary conferences held at some centers where a group of physicians look at your records, discuss your individual case, share their opinions with the group and make treatment recommendations as a team. If you have access to this type of conference, or group of physicians practicing as a team, this may serve as your second opinion.

Preparing for the Second Opinion Visit

When seeking a second opinion, you should clarify any questions you have. Make a list of your questions and concerns before the visit and take the list with you. Also, be sure that all requested lab and diagnostic test results are sent to the physician before your visit, to ensure that the needed information is available before the consultation. Call several days prior to your appointment and check to see if your records have arrived. The consulting physician will share his/her opinion with you and send recommendations to your physician, who can then take full advantage of the second opinion.

The most common benefit of a second opinion is to have peace of mind in knowing that you have gathered all the information that you need to make an informed decision. An informed decision allows you to go through your treatments knowing that this was the best treatment choice for you. Some women feel comfortable with their initial treatment options, feel their questions are answered sufficiently and feel no need for a second opinion. This is very acceptable. Seeking a second opinion is an individual decision and one that needs to be made according to your needs.

Remember

🕊 A second opinion is your opportunity to gather all the information you may need to experience peace of mind about your surgical and treatment decisions.

🕊 Be sure all your reports are sent prior to your visit and make a written list of all questions you need answered.

🕊 If the thought of a second opinion creates anxiety for you, it is not a good idea.

Reconstructive Surgery

Even though you are losing a breast or a part of a breast to surgery, you have the option to have your body image restored through plastic surgery. Breast reconstruction has made a big difference both physically and emotionally for many women who have undergone surgery for breast cancer. Some have immediate reconstruction at the time of initial breast surgery. They feel that reconstruction will help bring back their feminine silhouette and alleviate the necessity of a prosthesis. Others wait until their treatments for breast cancer have been completed. Some women choose never to have reconstruction.

If you feel that you would like to have your breast reconstructed, talk to your surgeon **prior** to your surgery. You may want to consult a reconstructive surgeon prior to your surgery, even if you plan to have the procedure performed after your treatments. Your surgeon or clinic can provide you with names of reconstructive surgeons who are competent in this field.

A decision to have reconstruction requires a lot of research and discussion. Remember, part of gaining control over your cancer is knowing all the options that are available to you and choosing those that best meet your needs.

Types of Reconstruction

There are many types of procedures available today which use implants or one's own body tissue to reconstruct your breast. Types of implants may be saline water filled or from other synthetic material, with variations of both available. Implants are usually placed under your chest muscle. Muscle from your abdomen or back or body fat may also be used to reconstruct your breast. Decisions as to which type of surgery would give you the best cosmetic results depend on:

- ◆ Your physical makeup (size of your breast, degree of sagging)

- ◆ Type of surgery (mastectomy or lumpectomy)

- ◆ Treatments given for your cancer (prior radiation therapy to the chest area may not allow some types of reconstruction to be performed)

- ◆ Your general health (example: a smoker may be a poor candidate for some types of surgery)

- ◆ Your preference for enlargement or reduction of the other breast during surgery

- ◆ Your personal goal and motivation for reconstruction

A woman is never too old for reconstructive surgery if she is in good health. **Health problems that may cause concern and limit surgical options include advanced diabetes mellitus, a recent heart attack or stroke or a history of severe, chronic lung disease.** Only a physician can evaluate the risks for your desired surgical decisions.

Ask your physician or clinic for reconstruction information that explains the surgical procedures and lists all the advantages and disadvantages. The American Cancer Society's **Reach To Recovery** coordinator can give you names of women who have had reconstructive surgery and who may be available to discuss their experiences with you.

Some of the advantages and disadvantages of immediate and delayed reconstruction are listed below. **Ask your reconstructive surgeon for additional comments.**

Advantages of Reconstruction
- Restores feminine body image
- No prosthesis or special bras have to be purchased and worn
- Can wear any clothing, including swimsuits and low-neck attire
- Can go braless
- Do not have the daily reminder of breast surgery (in the form of a prosthesis)
- Psychologically beneficial in allowing most women to adjust better to the disease

Disadvantages of Reconstruction
- Physical recovery from surgery will require more time, and you will experience a greater amount of pain
- Expense–some insurance companies may not cover all of the costs
- Increased potential for infection or surgical complications due to the more complex surgery

Immediate Versus Delayed Reconstruction

Advantages of Immediate Reconstruction
- One surgery experience, requiring only one anesthetic (being put to sleep)
- Lower cost than two separate surgeries
- Reduced recovery time in comparison to two separate surgeries
- Body image does not suffer as great a change as has been associated with mastectomy alone
- Psychologically, there **may** be some better adaptation

Disadvantages of Immediate Reconstruction
- More physical discomfort and longer recovery time after surgery, when emotions are at highest anxiety levels (much longer surgery if body tissues are used and slightly longer if implants are used)
- Increased potential for infection or surgical complications which could delay treatments for your cancer

36

Advantages of Delayed Reconstruction
- Time to carefully study reconstruction methods and talk to patients who have experienced varying procedures
- Time to carefully select reconstructive surgeon and seek several consultations if needed
- Psychologically less anxious over cancer experience at time of reconstructive surgery
- No delay in treatments (chemotherapy or radiation) because of infection or surgical complications from surgery
- Women with delayed reconstructed breasts may be happier than women who had immediate reconstruction because they experienced the inconvenience of having to wear a prosthesis and inability to go braless (thus their expectations were not as great.)

Disadvantages of Delayed Reconstruction
- Need for a second major surgery
- Higher cost because of second major surgery (anesthesia, surgery room, etc.)
- Cost of purchasing a prosthesis and special bras
- Inconvenience of having to wear a prosthesis until reconstructive surgery
- Temporarily unable to go braless or wear some low-cut clothing
- Procedure may fall into another deductible calendar year, requiring deductibles to be met for a second time. (Some insurance providers will not pay for a prosthesis and reconstruction. Only one option for restoring body image may be covered in a policy. Check your insurance policy.)
- Psychological distress from having to deal with an altered body image while waiting on reconstructive surgery

If you are considering reconstruction, make an appointment for a consultation with a plastic surgeon and discuss openly your feelings about the different procedures that may be used. (Questions on page 165.) After looking closely at your history, recommended surgical procedure (mastectomy or lumpectomy) and treatment recommendations (chemotherapy or radiation therapy), the surgeon will take into account your desired reconstructive surgery outcome, and a recommendation will be made for you.

Often women fear that reconstruction may hide or prevent the detection of recurrence of cancer in the breast area. There is **no** evidence of any kind that breast reconstruction causes cancer to grow or recur. Because the breast implant is usually placed beneath the chest wall muscles, there is little difficulty in detecting an early local recurrence. This fear should not be a concern in making your decision.

Questions You May Wish to Ask Your Reconstructive Surgeon

- What type of surgery do you recommend for me?
- Do you suggest the use of my own body tissue or an implant?
- What kind of implants do you recommend? Will they be placed under the muscle?
- What are the risks and benefits of this surgery?
- Can I see photographs and talk to some of your patients?
- What can I expect to look like after surgery?
- Will you reconstruct my nipple and areola?
- How much feeling (sensation) will I have in my reconstructed breast?
- How will my breast feel when touched (soft, firm)?
- Will this surgery cause me to have additional scars?
- How many surgical procedures will my reconstruction require?
- How long will I be in surgery for each of these procedures?
- How long will I be in the hospital for each procedure?
- How often will I need a return appointment with you?
- How long will it take to complete the reconstruction process?
- How long before I can return to work or normal activities after each procedure?
- How much will it cost, and how much should my insurance cover?

Remember

- Reconstruction is an option that all breast surgery patients need to know about, but not a procedure that all patients necessarily need to have.

- If all of this information overwhelms you, you do not have to make a decision now. Reconstruction can be performed at a later date, even years later. Make decisions based on what you feel best meets your needs.

The Role of the Oncologist

An oncologist, an internal medicine physician, specializes in the treatment of cancer. Your surgeon may have an oncologist evaluate you for cancer treatment before or after your surgery. It is very important that you have a good relationship with your oncologist if you are to receive other treatments in addition to your surgery. There will be a need for a great deal of interaction between you and the oncologist during the time you are receiving treatments. You should feel comfortable asking questions and participating in treatment decisions with your oncologist. The types of treatments that oncologists use consist of chemotherapy, immunotherapy or hormonal therapy. You may be referred to a radiation oncologist for radiation therapy. If you need further treatment, your oncologist will usually lead the treatment team after you are dismissed by your surgeon. Refer to Chapter 9 for a complete discussion on the role of the oncologist, chemotherapy and hormonal therapy. (Questions located on page 177.)

The Role of the Radiation Oncologist

A radiation oncologist is a physician who specializes in using radiation (x-ray) therapy to treat diseases. If your physician feels that radiation therapy could kill any remaining cancer cells in your body, you will be referred to a radiation oncologist. Most breast conserving surgeries are followed by radiation therapy. If you are having radiation therapy, it will be helpful to have a consultation with the radiation oncologist **before** your surgery. Refer to Chapter 9 for a full discussion of radiation therapy and the questions you may wish to ask during your consultation. (Questions located on page 179.)

Remember

❧ The selection of an oncologist is one of the most important treatment decisions you will make. Select a physician who allows you to ask questions, provides you with the information you need about your treatments and allows you to become a partner in recovery.

Refer to the tear-out worksheets, "Questions About Surgery," "Reconstructive Surgeon's Questions," "Personal Health Care Directory" and "Personal Treatment Record," located at the back of the book.

As Survivors,
we remember that even horrible losses
can be transformed into learning.
We decide, even in the midst of our pain,
to learn from our loss. We move from
the question of "Why me," to
"Now that this has happened, what
shall I do about it?"

Chapter 7

The Surgical Experience

"I had the normal fear of adjusting to the loss of my breast,
but by now I was more angry than afraid.
My worst nightmare had become a reality."

~ Harriett Barrineau, survivor

Preparation for Surgery

Prior to your surgery you will need to have a pre-admission physical assessment which is usually performed in the hospital where your surgery will take place. Lab work includes a profile of your blood components and body chemistry, urinalysis, chest x-ray, electrocardiogram and any other tests your physician may feel necessary. **Remember to take your insurance card or policy when going for this assessment**. If you have a living will or any special instructions, take them with you to be attached to your chart the day of surgery. It is now customary for everyone entering a hospital to be asked if they have a living will before any admission. This is asked of all patients and has nothing to do with your type of treatment or diagnosis. Also, take a list of any medications, prescription or nonprescription, that you regularly take.

A registered nurse will conduct an interview asking questions about your physical and medical history. You will be asked dates of previous surgeries or major illnesses and to list any allergies that you have experienced. Don't dismiss any detail as too insignificant or embarrassing to mention. It is better that the medical team be aware than be surprised by some complication. Tell the nurse or physician if you are under the care of another specialist, such as a cardiologist or pulmonologist, prior to your surgery. Be sure that your surgeon is aware of their names and telephone numbers. This assessment usually requires from one to two hours.

You will be given instructions about any special preparations before surgery. For example, you will be told not to eat or drink after midnight the day of your surgery and to stop smoking as long before surgery as possible. **Ask the nurse if you are to take any of your**

41

regular medications the morning of surgery. The time you should arrive before your surgery and the scheduled time of your surgery will be provided during your pre-admission visit. Ask if there are any restrictions on the number of people allowed to wait in the surgical waiting room. Request the telephone number to this waiting room to provide for other family members or friends.

Blood transfusions are rarely needed with lumpectomy and mastectomy surgeries. Occasionally, some types of reconstruction may require that blood be available if needed. If you are planning reconstructive surgery, you may want to consult with your surgeon about donating your own blood before you are hospitalized. Information on how to arrange to have your blood collected and stored can be provided by your doctor.

Packing for Your Hospital Visit
When packing your suitcase to take to the hospital, you will need to remember:

- Personal hygiene items: comb, brush, toothbrush, toothpaste, deodorant, makeup and shampoo

- Robe and gown or pajamas (two to three changes—better if they are front-opening)

- Undergarments

- Bedroom shoes

- Reading material

- Telephone numbers of family and friends

- Pencil and note paper

- Pillow to elevate your arm in hospital and to use with your seatbelt on your ride home

- Clothes to wear home (Some women find that large, soft sweatshirts are comfortable. You don't have to wear a bra, and they conceal any surgical drain that may be in place.)

It will be psychologically and physically helpful to have someone plan to be with you on the day of surgery. A trained nurse is not necessary because mastectomy and lumpectomy surgeries are usually relatively simple and do not involve extensive assistance after surgery. A family member or friend will be able to assist you and make this time more comfortable (for example, by helping you to the bathroom or getting you something to drink).

Informed Consent

Sometime before your surgery you will be asked to sign an informed consent. Consent forms will also be presented before chemotherapy, radiation therapy or reconstructive surgery for your signature. Your physician or an assistant will explain to you the procedures that will be performed and the possible risks involved. This will occur before sedation is given. **Read**

the consent form carefully. It will contain the following information:

- ◆ Type of surgery and treatment you will receive
- ◆ Name of the doctor who will perform the surgery or treatment
- ◆ Risks of the surgery or treatment
- ◆ Advantages of the surgery or treatment
- ◆ Identification of any experimental treatments
- ◆ Benefits of the surgery or treatment
- ◆ When the treatment will begin and end

By signing this form you will acknowledge that you understand and have no other questions. Discuss with the surgeon what type of post-operative pain management will be used and if the medication will be given on request. If you do not understand and would like more information, this is the time to request it.

The Day of Your Surgery

On the day of surgery you will need to report to the surgery area at the assigned time. Do not wear jewelry (watches, rings, earrings) or contact lenses. Eyeglasses may be needed to read and sign admission forms. Dental bridges or false teeth can be worn and removed just prior to your surgery. The nurse will place them in a special storage container during surgery and they will be made available to you as soon as you are alert. Do not bring money, credit cards or a check book. Leave these with family members or at home.

You will be interviewed by your anesthesiologist (the physician who administers the anesthesia) before going to surgery. Some anesthesiologists may prefer an interview prior to the day of surgery. Your medical history will be reviewed before surgery. Inform your nurse if any changes in your health have occurred since the initial assessment (cold, fever, diarrhea, etc.).

You will be taken to a room where you will undress and begin preparing for surgery. You will be given a medication to keep you calm. Your underarm area will be shaved. An intravenous needle to be used for medications and fluids will be inserted into the arm opposite the surgical site.

After entering the surgical suite you will be positioned upon a surgical table. A cuff will be placed on your arm to monitor your blood pressure, a device placed on your finger to measure the oxygen in your blood and an electrocardiogram machine hooked up to monitor your heart. The surgeon will cleanse a large area surrounding the site of the surgical incision. You will be given your anesthesia some time during this process. After you are asleep, you will have a tube placed in your throat to facilitate your breathing. Your surgery will then be performed.

When the surgical procedure is completed you will be transferred to a post-anesthesia (recovery) room. Your blood pressure, oxygen level and heart rate will be monitored while in this room. Usually, you are in recovery for two or more hours. When you are awake and your vital signs are in normal range, you will be transferred to your room or allowed to return home. Some lumpectomy and mastectomy patients are allowed to return home the same day. If you are to leave the same day, you will be transferred to an outpatient recovery room and monitored until the health care team determines that you are in stable condition and are physically able to travel home. You will be given discharge instructions at this time. Refer to page 50 for the questions to ask about your care at home.

You will have a bandage on your chest and may have one or more bulb drains at the surgical site to reduce accumulation of fluid, which can place pressure on your incision. If at any time you notice that your bandage feels wet, notify your nurse or follow your discharge instructions if you are at home. If you see bright red blood coming through your bandage, notify your nurse, or if at home, call your physician's office as soon as possible. Some types of surgery may not require a drain. If you have a drain, at first the drainage will be bright red from blood, but it will gradually change to a lighter color over the next few days. The length of time your drain remains in place varies according to where the drain is placed and the amount of fluid that accumulates in the drain. Ask your physician her/his plan for drain removal.

Discomfort After Surgery

Most women are surprised at the small amount of pain they experience after their surgery. Pain medication has been ordered by the physician to control any pain you experience, but if hospitalized, you must request it from the nurse. If you have pain, use your nurse call button to let your nurse know so the medication can be administered.

The pain experienced after breast surgery has been described by women as a discomfort in the breast area, accompanied by numbness or tingling in the arm. Others say that they felt pain in the breast that was removed which felt like a heaviness or sensations from the nipple. Doctors call this **phantom pain** because, even though the breast is gone, the brain perceives the sensation of pain from the remaining nerves. Some of the nerves on the chest wall may be irritated or cut during the surgical procedure, and this causes a feeling of numbness across the chest. Most women state that most discomfort is under the arm where the lymph nodes were removed. This pain often radiates down the arm, and you may feel as if needles or pins are sticking you. The arm may also feel numb. The numbness is not unusual, and the sensation may or may not improve in the coming months. Incisional pain is usually over in about a week to ten days, and the referred sensations will improve as arm mobility is restored. The surgical staff's goal is that you experience the minimum amount of pain, and they will provide you with the amount of medication required to keep you comfortable.

You may also have a slight headache or nausea from the residual anesthesia after you awake. This is not unusual and often may be caused from the long period of time you have been without food. Resume eating by taking fluids first, adding light foods and then progressing to your normal diet as you desire. Nausea can be aggravated by heavy foods.

Your throat may feel sore from the tube inserted during surgery. Soreness in the back or shoulder area is very common because of the position you were required to be in during surgery. This soreness will last for several days. Whatever you may experience, tell your nurse so you can be kept as comfortable as possible.

Personal Hygiene After Surgery

For the next few days you may need to take a sponge bath to keep your dressing dry. Ask your doctor when you have permission for a shower or a tub bath. The dressing should always be kept dry. You can tape a plastic bag or plastic wrap over the area while you bathe. If at any time the dressing becomes wet, you need to have it changed.

Your physician will tell you when you can use your surgical arm to shampoo your hair. Do not use deodorant under the surgical arm for the first six weeks. Perspiration odor is unusual because of glands removed during surgery. However, you may wipe the area with an alcohol pad or peroxide if you feel a need to cleanse the area. Avoid allowing the alcohol to run into the surgical area and cause stinging.

Post-Surgical Arm Care

Your surgical arm will be sore but you need to continue to use your hand to feed yourself, comb your hair and wash your face. This will help the soreness to improve. Keeping your surgical arm propped up on a pillow, above the level of your heart, will assist in preventing fluid accumulation and swelling in the arm, reducing the pain. Plan to elevate your arm for 45 minutes, twice a day for the first six weeks after surgery. But **do not lift** anything heavy (over 1-2 pounds) or **begin** any **exercises** until your **physician gives you permission**.

Rest After Surgery

The first days after surgery you may feel sleepy and tired from the anesthesia and all the stress that accumulated prior to the surgery. If you don't feel up to having many visitors, ask your nurse to place a "No Visitors" sign on your door or have family members receive guests.

You may also take the telephone off the hook in the hospital or turn the ringer off at home. Or you may ask family members or friends to speak to visitors or answer the telephone when you need rest. If hospitalized, ask for medications to keep you comfortable. Most pain and nausea medications have to be requested by you. If you are recovering at home, follow your physician's instructions on the amount and time to take your medications. If you do not have pain relief or nausea relief, contact your physician so that appropriate changes can be made.

The Surgical Incision

Your first dressing change will occur before you leave the hospital unless you have outpatient surgery—in which case, you will return to the physician's office. Some women report it was difficult to view the incision for the first time, but afterwards they were glad they did. Viewing the incision may also be difficult for your mate. Many women feel that viewing the incision together the first time was helpful in their future adjustment. Postponing the viewing does not make it easier or help either of you.

It is important that you observe the incision area carefully at this time to learn what is normal for the scar area. This will help as you monitor the incision for changes after you return home. A mastectomy scar is one long scar. You may have sutures or staples to close the incision. A lumpectomy will have an incision on the breast and another under the arm where lymph nodes lymph nodes were removed. Your doctor or nurse will provide instructions at this time on how and when to change the dressing and changes to report to the medical staff. It will be helpful if a family member is present during instructions to help you understand and assist you with your dressing or drains.

Care of Your Dressing

The goal of care for your incision is to keep a clean, dry dressing in place and monitor the area for changes that might indicate an infection. Types of dressings vary with physicians, but all dressings need to remain dry. A wet dressing will set up an environment for bacteria to breed and may cause an infection. If you have a dressing and it becomes damp, follow your physician's instructions for changing the dressing. Sutures or staples are removed five to ten days later in the doctor's office.

Your surgeon or nurse will discuss care of your dressing prior to discharge. It may help to have a family member assist with dressing changes because of the soreness you will experience and the difficulty of working on your own chest. It is helpful if they are present when dressing changes are discussed. Ask your nurse for dressing supplies to take home. Follow special orders from your physician for dressing changes. If you do not receive orders, the steps to follow for changing a dressing are listed below:

- Gather all dressing supplies: paper bag, dressing (gauze), tape, scissors, alcohol wipes or gauze pads
- Wash your hands
- Prepare tape strips
- Remove the old dressing
- Note the color, odor and amount of drainage on dressing
- Dispose of the old dressing in a paper bag
- Wash your hands thoroughly with soap
- Observe incision carefully
- Wipe off any old blood or tape residue with an alcohol wipe. Always start wiping near the incision and wipe away from the incision, **not** back over it.
- Place clean dressing on the area and tape it into place
- Dispose of paper bag containing old dressing
- Wash your hands

Monitoring Your Incision

When changing your dressing, observe first the old bandage for signs of drainage. Normal drainage is a blood-tinged, watery discharge. Discharge that is thick and yellowish to greenish in color may indicate infection. Often this type of discharge will have a foul odor. If you notice this occurring, notify your physician.

Carefully observe the incision site. An increase in redness, swelling and signs of discharge anywhere along the incision line may indicate a potential infection. Call your physician, and ask for instructions. Often, early intervention may require a local antibiotic to the area.

Ask your physician when you may take a shower or tub bath and use soap and water on the area. Some physicians allow showers first because of the constant flow of clean water over the incision. After your bath/shower, pat the area dry and protect it with a soft dressing or covering to prevent irritation and rubbing by your clothing. Some find that a soft tee shirt or a long-line cotton sports bra, which is sold in department stores, serves this purpose.

It is important **not** to allow any powder, deodorant, lotions or perfumes to come in contact with the surgical incision site. These products should be avoided for four to six weeks past surgery or until the site has healed completely. Again, perspiration odor will not be a problem under the surgical arm because of the removal of glands in the underarm area. However, if you wish, you may wipe the area with an alcohol wipe or peroxide to further cleanse after your bath.

Care of Your Drain Bulbs

Instructions will also be given on how to care for your drain(s) if you have them. Drains are inserted to collect fluid accumulation at the surgery site and to reduce swelling and pain. The tubing is anchored to your tissue during surgery. At the end of the tubing is a soft plastic bulb with a plug that allows the fluid to be emptied.

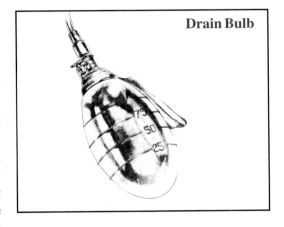

Drain Bulb

The fluid that accumulates in the drain bulb is a mixture of blood cells and lymphatic fluid. During surgery, the lymphatic system vessels are cut, causing the microscopic vessels to empty their fluid into the area. The drainage will be dark red at first because of the large amount of blood cells in the area. It will gradually change to pink-tinged and finally to a yellow, straw color. The amount of drainage varies, and there is no way to predict how much drainage any woman will accumulate. Some women have large amounts and others have a minimal amount. Gradually, these small vessels seal themselves off, and the fluid stops accumulating. The time this takes varies among women. Neither body size nor age seems to determine the amount. However, the amount of drainage during the first 24 hours often predicts the accumulation volume later.

Physicians remove the drains when the amount of drainage is reduced to between 20 to 50 ccs ($^1/_2$-$1^1/_2$ ounces or 4 to 10 teaspoons) per drain, per 24 hours. Some women have very little drainage and have their drain(s) removed within the first week. Others may need their drain(s) for several weeks and, occasionally, longer. If the drain(s) are removed too soon, the fluid can accumulate under the skin, forming a **seroma** (collection of fluid), and become painful by putting pressure on the surgical site. Neither the amount of fluid produced nor the length of time required to have drains has anything to do with your cancer. Fluid and drains are only related to the amount of fluid your lymph system produces.

Care of your drains will be discussed by your nurse. It is important not to allow the drains to hang loosely. **Always secure them to your clothing and empty them when they become heavy.** The first day may require emptying every several hours. Later, twice a day will be sufficient. Pressure caused from a heavy drain, not pinned to your clothing and pulling on your incision site, can cause **pain and scar formation at the drain insertion site.** The scar will heal but will be thick and have an uneven appearance. Be careful not to allow drains to drop away from your body.

Emptying and Recording Your Drainage

Empty drains when they become heavy or over half-filled with fluid. When your drainage has decreased to a small amount, empty twice a day.

- If you have more than one drain, place a piece of tape on each, and mark them with numbers (drain 1 or drain 2). Refer to the amounts emptied, and record by number designation.
- Gather your supplies: a drain record (found in the back of this book), pencil or pen and a measuring cup.
- Open one drain by removing the plug in the drain bulb, and empty drainage into a measuring cup.
- Squeeze the air out of the empty bulb and keep the bulb squeezed as flat as possible as you replug the drain. This compression of the bulb encourages the flow of fluid from the surgical site into the bulb.
- If any of the drainage spilled onto the outside of the bulb, wipe it off with a damp cloth using soap and water or an alcohol wipe.
- Secure the bulb by pinning it to clothing or placing it into a surgical drainage bag holder. Do not allow bulb to hang freely.
- Measure the drainage in the cup.
- Observe the color of the drainage. If you begin noticing that the fluid has changed color, becoming a darker red or appears to have fresh blood reappearing after the color had changed to a light pink, contact your physician and inform him/her of the change.
- Empty the drainage into the toilet and flush. You do not save the drainage.
- Wash your hands with soap and water.
- Record drainage under the appropriate column, documenting the time emptied.
- If you have a second drain, repeat the process.

◆ Take the written drainage record to the surgeon on your return visit. An accurate record will assist the physician in determining when to remove your drain(s). (A tear-out record sheet to record your drainage at home is located on page 171 of this workbook.)

Potential Post-Surgical Problems

Fluid Leakage at Drain Site

Occasionally, a small amount of fluid will leak from the insertion site of the tubing. This is not dangerous. However, you should apply a sterile dressing and change the dressing when it becomes damp. Do not allow a wet dressing to remain in place. The dressing should be changed as often as needed to prevent irritation and breakdown of the skin. A wet dressing will allow bacteria to grow. If large amounts of fluid begin leaking from the site, call your surgeon or nurse and ask for instructions.

Clogged Drains

Bulb drains may clog because of the formation of small clots in the tubing. This is not an unusual occurrence. If you notice that there is no fluid in the bulb, check the tubing for a possible blockage caused by a clot. If a clot is found or if your drain has stopped draining, perform the following steps to reopen drainage:

◆ Wash your hands with soap and water.

◆ Gently squeeze the area in which the clot is located to dislodge it.

◆ After squeezing the clot, begin near the insertion site on your chest and squeeze downward the entire length of the tubing toward the drainage bulb. Do not pull on the tubing. Repeat the process several times, squeezing the entire length of the drainage tubing.

◆ Secure drains to prevent hanging loosely.

◆ Monitor the drain bulb for fluid accumulation. After several hours if no drainage has accumulated, notify your physician for further instructions.

Monitoring Drains for Infection

It is very rare for infections to occur with bulb drains. However, if you notice the insertion site begins to have an increased redness, discharge of pus (thick yellowish or greenish fluid) or foul odor, then notify your physician of these changes. **The main prevention for infection is to keep the area clean and dry.**

Drain Removal

Drains are removed by the surgeon during an office visit. Women report a pulling feeling with a moderate amount of pain lasting for a few seconds when the drain is removed. A small bandage is placed over the drain removal site. This site will also need to be monitored for infection for the next several days. Any increase in redness, swelling, discharge or pain should be reported to your surgeon's office.

Seromas

Before or after your drains are removed, if you have a painful accumulation of fluid at the incision site, below the incision site or in the underarm area, notify your physician. This fluid accumulation is called a **seroma**. The accumulation of fluid feels much like water in a balloon when it forms under the skin. If a seroma continues to increase in size and puts pressure on your incision, it can become painful.

Seromas are the most common complication after surgery. Painful seromas may require the withdrawal of the fluid from the area using a small needle and an empty syringe by the physician. This procedure is performed in the physician's office. Withdrawal of the fluid is relatively painless, and aspiration of the fluid relieves the pain. However, as with any invasive procedure, the potential for infection increases. You will need to monitor the area and report any redness, swelling or pain to your physician. Occasionally, the fluid will continue to accumulate requiring several aspirations by the surgeon. This fluid accumulation has **nothing** to do with your cancer. It is related to lymphatic fluid accumulation in the area.

Hospital Discharge Instructions

Prior to leaving the hospital, your nurse will provide you with verbal and written instructions concerning your care and a list of symptoms that might occur and need to be reported to the doctor. During your hospitalization, it may be helpful to write down any questions as they occur. When your doctor makes the final hospital visit, you may want to be prepared to clarify the following:

- If you do not remember what you were told about your surgery or diagnosis the day you had surgery, ask for clarification.
- What activities can I do with my surgical arm until my next appointment?
- Are there any special exercises or recommendations regarding use of my arm?
- Are the numbness, tingling or sensations I am experiencing temporary or permanent?
- What medications will I take for pain?
- What kind of pain is normal after my type of surgery?
- Will I be given any prescriptions for medication to take home?
- Do I resume previous medications (especially estrogen-type medications)?
- When can I shampoo my hair?
- When can I shower or take a tub bath?
- When can I remove my bandage?

◆ When can I drive?

◆ When and how do I make my next appointment?

◆ Will I be referred to any other doctors or have any other treatments? If so, when will I see these doctors?

◆ When will my pathology report be available?

◆ Is there anything special that I can do to ensure a speedy recovery?

Ask your nurse to write down any appointment dates or names of doctors to whom you will be referred for further evaluation concerning treatment. Inform your doctor or nurse early if you have a physical limitation that would prevent you from being able to manage at home. A home health service or aide to assist you for a short period of time can be ordered before you leave the hospital. Ask for a telephone number that you can call after you return home if you have any questions regarding your discharge instructions. Some hospitals will provide you with supplies necessary for your dressing changes at home. Ask your nurse about dressing supplies. (Discharge questions on page 173.)

Seatbelt Use After Surgery
On your ride home from the hospital it will be helpful if you have a small pillow to place over your chest and the area of your incision so that you will be able to wear your seat belt in the car. Sudden stops can cause pain and potential injury to new mastectomy or lumpectomy surgical sites from the sudden pressure of a seat belt. The protection provided by the pillow can prevent this type of injury or discomfort and make the wearing of your seat belt more comfortable. Using the pillow for protection when wearing a seat belt is helpful for the first several weeks after your surgery if the seat belt crosses your incision.

Recovering at Home

Your discharge instructions from the hospital give you information as to when you need to call the physician, how to manage your drains and how to change your bandage. Recovery from surgery for breast cancer usually requires two to three weeks. Discomfort in the incisional area(s) will improve daily, usually resolving within ten days. In five to six weeks most women report that they have resumed their normal activities. Remember, we are all different. Listen to the cues from your body, rest when needed and resume your normal activities when you feel up to them.

Your incision will change color as it heals; this is normal. Initially the scar will be red and raised for several months past surgery. The redness is caused by the additional blood flow to promote healing in the area. The redness and thickness of the scar will subside over the next one to two years, and the area will become less obvious and very faint in color.

Plan to begin your exercise program to restore your normal range of motion to the surgical arm as soon as the physician gives you permission. Report any problems you have performing the exercises to your physician.

It is important that you keep your follow-up appointments with the surgeon. You will be monitored for proper healing and return of proper range of motion in your surgical arm. Your remaining breast will also be closely checked.

Uncommon Post-Surgical Problems

Most women have very few problems after breast surgery. However, there are some uncommon problems which may arise from the surgical procedure and of which you may need to be aware. These problems have nothing to do with the cancer but are due to the surgery.

Phlebitis

Occasionally some women will have very little pain immediately after their surgery only to experience a pain which begins days later. The pain may radiate down the arm, usually to the elbow, but sometimes to the wrist. This occurs when the basilic vein in the arm has become inflamed after the surgery, called **phlebitis**. This inflammation, which is not serious, causes pain which can be helped with an analgesic such as aspirin. This is not common and will resolve in several days to a week. This pain may limit your ability to perform your exercises. Inform your physician if this should occur.

Sensitive Surgical Site

Another problem a very small percent of women experience is **sensitive skin** in the surgical area. After surgery, even clothing is painful if it touches the incision area. If this occurs, inform your physician. Occasionally, the nerves in the area are super sensitive and will need a procedure called "desensitization" to decrease the sensation. This procedure is performed by a physical therapist. The therapist can instruct you on the procedure to perform at home if needed, and this then becomes part of your daily exercise routine.

Frozen Shoulder

Failure to use your arm **after** the physician has given you permission to begin exercises to restore normal range of motion can result in a condition called a "**frozen shoulder**." This condition causes pain and inability to move the shoulder freely; however, it is a rare occurrence. Any complication which can keep you from proceeding with your exercise program should be brought to the surgeon's attention. Restoring full range of motion is accomplished by gradually increasing the movements of the arm (using exercises such as the ones in Chapter 10).

Remember

> Surgery for breast cancer is usually not very painful physically, but it may be very painful emotionally.

> Ask your health care team for what you need to make this time as easy as possible for you; additional information or instructions, pain medication, privacy, access to a chaplain, etc. You are employing them to meet your needs.

> Tell your support partner, family or friends what you need from them during this time. Be honest.

> Do not hesitate to call your physician if any problems arise when you return home.

Use the time of your surgery to rekindle your emotions and energy. Rest when needed. Be good to yourself. Think about any changes you would like to make in your life. At no other time in life will people give you as much permission to make changes.

What is it you have always wanted to do—a new hobby, go on a trip, take a class, get a pet, start an exercise program? You decide what will give you the most happiness and GO FOR IT. Breast cancer is not a valid excuse to forgo planning for events and activities that will bring you happiness. Plan your exciting new future! Use breast cancer as the reason and not the excuse!

Refer to the tear-out worksheets, "Bulb Drain Record" and "Hospital Discharge Instructions," located at the back of the book.

*As Survivors,
we find people who will
help—friends, family, peers,
support groups, role models,
professional helpers, neighbors,
authors, treatment programs, wig
or prostheses makers—all who give
good advice of various and sundry
sorts to make our journey
a little easier.*

Chapter 8

Prosthesis Selection After Surgery

*"The day I was fitted with my prosthesis was a major step
in my road to recovery. For the first time in weeks,
I began to feel that life just might return to normal again."*

~ Harriett Barrineau, survivor

Restoring your body image after breast surgery is an important part of recovery. A prosthesis is a form molded as a breast and is worn inside your bra. Prostheses vary from a soft fiber filling placed in your bra to a custom-made form of your breast. Some women prefer not to leave the hospital without a way to appear balanced in their body image. To make this possible, a temporary soft prosthesis, a fabric form which can be filled with fiber filling to match the size of the remaining breast, can be placed into a bra. When the incision is healed a permanent prosthesis can be selected.

Temporary Prosthesis

Many patients receive a visit by an American Cancer Society's **Reach To Recovery** volunteer. The volunteer, a woman who has had breast cancer, will visit you in the hospital or at your home, bringing many helpful ideas for your recovery. Some units provide the Reach To Recovery volunteer with a soft bra and a soft temporary prosthesis for you to wear the first couple of weeks, if you so desire. Ask your surgeon if you will receive a visit before or while you are in the hospital and if your local unit provides this service.

If you desire to purchase your own temporary prosthesis, check with your local prosthesis fitter. You can find the names located in your phone book under Prosthetic Devices, or you can ask your surgeon's staff for recommendations. Prosthetic shops specialize in custom forms, and you can purchase soft, front-opening bras and a form you fill with a soft fiber to match the size of your remaining breast. Some women have found it helpful to purchase these items before their surgery. This allows them to restore their body image soon after a mastectomy and before they can be fitted with a prosthesis.

Wearing a Bra

Women who have breast conserving surgeries (lumpectomies) usually are more comfortable with a bra immediately after surgery to prevent movement of the remaining breast tissue. A well-fitting bra can prevent much discomfort experienced because of excessive movement of the breast tissues. Sleeping in the bra can also be helpful.

Mastectomy patients often find that a bra right after surgery is uncomfortable and tends to rub the incision area. They feel more comfortable braless while wearing a soft cotton, large sweatshirt until their incision heals. Some find a man's cotton tee shirt is a good choice and can be worn under their clothing. A sports, cotton exercise bra, found in any department store, is comfortable for some. Others are comfortable wearing a lightweight bra with a temporary prosthesis of fiber filling. Some choose to go braless at home and wear their lightweight bra and prosthesis when going out. You be the judge of what suits your needs best, either a soft bra or braless. **However, do not wear any bra which rubs or causes irritation to your incision while it is healing.** Reconstructive surgery patients need to ask their reconstructive surgeon for recommendations on wearing a bra during the weeks following surgery.

The lightweight temporary prosthesis presents a problem—the bra rides up and causes the prosthesis to be higher on the chest wall. This can be corrected by anchoring the bra to other undergarments (panties) with a piece of elastic which is attached by snaps or Velcro, pinned or sewn on, to hold the bra down in position. Weights, such as those used in curtains and found in fabric shops, may also be sewn into the bra cup on the prosthesis side to add weight and prevent the riding up of the bra.

Mastectomy Bras

Special mastectomy bras are available, but many women prefer to purchase a prosthesis that fits in their favorite bra. This bra should **not** have **underwires** and must fit well. The fitter can help you decide if this is possible with your existing bras. She can show you how to create a pocket in which to place the prosthesis in order to prevent it from falling out.

Permanent Prosthesis Selection

When your incision has healed, usually four to six weeks following surgery, your physician will give you a prescription for a prosthesis, which allows you to file for insurance coverage for the prosthesis. Do not be fitted until your surgical site has healed. For some patients this may take longer.

When ready to shop for a prosthesis, it is best to make an appointment for a fitting with a trained prosthetic specialist. The specialist will help you decide on a prosthesis according to your breast size, the weight you need in a prosthesis and your life-style. Plan to go when you have time to look carefully at all she has to offer so you can find the prosthesis that best suits your needs. A fitting usually takes between one and two hours. When you go for your fitting, take or wear a close-fitting garment so that you can see what your body looks like with the prosthesis. Some women have found a man's cotton tee shirt is easily accessible. If possible, take a friend or your mate with you, someone who can see how the prosthesis looks and who will give you an honest opinion.

Types of Permanent Prostheses

Breast forms, like our breasts, come in many shapes and sizes. They may feel rubbery and very much like your own skin. They may be covered with a soft fabric, polyurethane or a silicone envelope. Some are filled with foam rubber, chemical gels, polyethylene material, polyurethane foam or silicone gel.

Like natural breasts, prostheses vary in weight, and their consistency varies from soft and pliable to relatively firm. They are also designed for the right and left side. Some have nipples that will appear much like your remaining breast. Forms are designed to fit into special pockets inside mastectomy bras to prevent the prosthesis from falling out.

There is also a model that attaches to your skin with an adhesive tape (much like Velcro) so that when you move, it moves. This model also prevents the riding up of the prosthesis in the bra, which is a problem for many women. If you feel this would be appropriate for your life-style, you may ask to try the adhesive and tape. Wear it for several days to be sure that you do not have an allergenic reaction. This prosthesis can be worn with your regular bras, and you can also go braless.

If you have reconstruction and do not have the nipple reconstructed, there are nipple prostheses. Women that have had segmental mastectomies or lumpectomies may need a prosthesis called an equalizer, which is designed to fill in the section of tissue removed from the breast.

Altering Clothing for Prostheses

You can also learn from the fitter how to alter your swimsuits for use with your prosthesis. Extremely lightweight forms are available for use with your nightgown or leisure clothes. Many clothing items such as sportswear, lingerie and swimsuits that accommodate a prosthesis are also sold in prosthetic shops. Some women buy silky, lacy camisoles and sew lightweight prostheses inside to wear under their nightclothes and when they do not want to put on their regular prosthesis.

What You Need to Know Before You Purchase a Prosthesis

It is important to ask your fitter the following questions about your prosthesis:

◆ How do I clean my prosthesis?

◆ Can I get it wet?

◆ How long will it take to dry?

◆ Does perspiration damage the prosthesis?

◆ Will pool chemicals cause any damage?

◆ Is there an exchange policy if I decide it does not meet my needs?

◆ How long should the prosthesis last?

◆ How much will my insurance provider pay toward the cost?

◆ Does my insurance company pay for mastectomy bras?

- If yes, how many bras will my insurance pay for at my initial purchase?
- How often will my insurance provider pay replacement costs of my prosthesis?
- How often will they pay for replacement bras?
- If I alter them, can I wear my regular bras with my selected prosthesis?
- Do you bill the provider for the cost, or do I pay and bill my provider?

What Prostheses Cost

Prices range from a few dollars for fiber filling up to around $350 for a permanent prosthesis. Most women spend around $250 for a prosthesis. Custom-made prostheses and prostheses that adhere to your body are more expensive. Bras range from 20 dollars up.

Most professional shops will assist you in finding out what your insurance company or Medicare will pay on your prosthesis and bras. **Some insurance policies state that they will only pay for a prosthesis or reconstruction.** If you plan to have reconstruction later, this may prevent the provider from covering the cost of your surgery if you file for the cost of a prosthesis. **Check your policy or call your provider if you plan for later reconstructive surgery.**

When You Cannot Afford a Prosthesis

If you cannot afford a prosthesis, some local **American Cancer Society** units have loan closets. Women who have had reconstruction may donate their prostheses to be given to other women who cannot afford one. Call your local American Cancer Society to ask if they provide this service.

The **Y-Me** organization has a Prosthesis and Wig Bank to provide women with financial needs a free breast prosthesis or a wig, if they have the appropriate size of prosthesis or color of wig available. A small handling charge is requested, and the product is mailed anywhere in the United States. The telephone number is listed in the resource section at the end of this book.

Ask your health care team if they know of any sources that assist women in the purchase of a prosthesis after surgery. Some local organizations may offer this type of support for patients who cannot afford to purchase needed prosthetic devices.

Remember

- Plan to shop for a prosthesis when you have time to carefully evaluate which breast form best suits your need. Make an appointment with a specialized fitter.

- Take someone with you who will be supportive and honest in helping you evaluate how it looks. Take a tee shirt or tight sweater to try on over the new form to see how it looks under clothing.

- Do not try to save a few dollars on a prosthesis you do not like or feel comfortable wearing. Restoring your body image is a very important part of recovery.

Refer to the tear-out worksheet, "Prosthesis Selection Questions," located at the back of the book.

*As Survivors,
we refuse to carry along old resentments,
grievances, axes to grind or remembered
injustices because we know that harbored
memories grow increasingly heavy and slow
our journey to recovery. Instead, we decide
not to waste our lives by permanently losing
ourselves in sorrow, defeat, anger, fear or guilt.
We lighten our recovery load by unloading
these energy drainers.*

Chapter 9

Post-Surgical Treatment Decisions

*"I was serious about wanting to know about breast cancer.
I wanted to be a part of my treatments.
I wanted to know what was being done and why."*
~ Harriett Barrineau, survivor

The preliminary pathology report you received after your biopsy contained much information about your cancer. A final pathology report will be prepared after your surgery. Your treatment plan is based on both the preliminary and the final biopsy report. From these two reports your physicians will determine which treatment is best suited for your individual case. The most common treatments are chemotherapy, radiation therapy or hormonal therapy. Your treatment may consist of one or more types of treatment. For some women, no further treatment may be needed, only close observation by the physician. A brief explanation of each type of treatment will be discussed. Your physician will provide you with specific information regarding your treatment plan.

Your Pathology Report

Because treatment decisions will be based on the pathology report on your tumor, it may be helpful to understand its importance in determining your treatment options. **However, it is not essential that you understand all of the following information. Some people feel that this is more information than they want to know. Feel free to skip this section.** It is included in case you need to have some questions about your pathology report clarified.

When your tumor was removed from your breast, it was sent to a pathology laboratory. There, a pathologist (a physician who specializes in diagnosing diseases from tissue samples) analyzed and issued a pathology report to your physician. This report will help your physicians determine if you need additional treatment. If additional treatment is needed, the pathology report will be used by the oncologist (a cancer specialist) to develop a treatment plan for your cancer. The pathology report will give information on the following aspects of your tumor.

61

Types of Breast Cancer

The most common types of breast cancer are listed below. There are also various other rare types of breast cancer and combinations of the following types.

- Infiltrating (invasive) ductal (approximately 54% of patients)
- In situ ductal (intraductal) (approximately 19%)
- Invasive lobular (approximately 5%)
- In situ lobular (approximately 2%)
- Medullary (approximately 6%)
- Mucinous (colloid, approximately 3%)
- Paget's disease with intraductal (approximately 1%)
- Paget's disease with invasive ductal (approximately 1%)

The remaining cancers occur in 1% or less:

- Tubular
- Adenocystic
- Papillary
- Inflammatory
- Scirrhous
- Carcinosarcoma
- Apocrine
- Squamous

Tumor Size

Tumor size is the largest dimension of the tumor. Results are reported in centimeters (cm) or millimeters (mm). (10 mm equals 1 cm. 1 cm equals 3/8 inch. 1 inch equals 2.5 cm.)

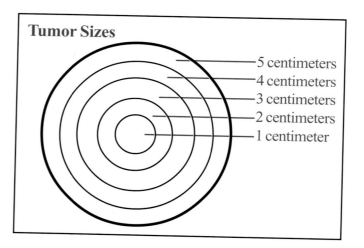

Tumor Sizes

- 5 centimeters
- 4 centimeters
- 3 centimeters
- 2 centimeters
- 1 centimeter

Margins

The margins describe the area surrounding a tumor, or if the entire tumor was removed it is how the margins relate to the tumor. If the tissue surrounding the tumor had **no** evidence of cancer cells, then the terms used will be "clear," "clean" or "uninvolved." If cancer is found in the margins, the terms may be "involved," or "residual cancer." If the pathologists were unable to make a definite statement, the term "indeterminate" may be used.

Tumor Shape

The report may also state the shape of the tumor as round or spherical (well circumscribed) or irregular shape (stellate, poorly circumscribed). The more irregular the shape of a tumor, the higher the potential to be aggressive.

Types of Cancer

- ◆ **In Situ Cancer**—Normal ducts and lobules are lined with one or more layers of cells in an orderly pattern. It is considered "in situ cancer" when cancer develops and grows in the duct or lobule where it began, but **does not** break through the cell wall. This type has a good prognosis.

- ◆ **Invasive (Infiltrating) Cancer**— Cancers that have broken through the wall of the duct or lobule and have begun to grow into surrounding tissues in the breast are considered invasive or infiltrating.

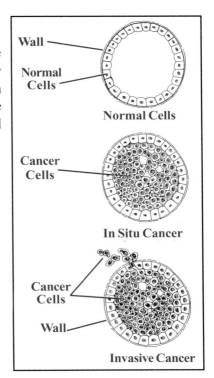

Normal Cells

In Situ Cancer

Invasive Cancer

Node Status

If surgery included lymph node removal, the report will state how many nodes were removed, a description of the area from which nodes came and how many nodes tested positive with cancer cells.

Grading of Tumor

The grading of cells is a microscopic examination describing the degree of change from the original, parent cell. This grading determines aggressiveness. Tumors are classified as:

- ◆ **Grade 1: Well differentiated tumors**—Less than 25% of cells are abnormal. Approximately 75% or more of the cells are very similar in appearance to the parent cell from which they evolved. They look similar, like sisters. Usually least aggressive.
- ◆ **Grade 2: Moderately differentiated tumors**—About 25 - 50% of cells are abnormal. Between 50 - 75 % of cells still resemble the parent cell. They are like first cousins. Term describes cells between the well and poorly differentiated stages.
- ◆ **Grade 3: Poorly differentiated cells**—Nearly 50 - 75% of cells are abnormal; 25 - 50 % of cells resemble the parent cell. Similar to third cousins. Usually aggressive.
- ◆ **Grade 4: Undifferentiated cells**—More than 75% of the cells are abnormal. Only 25% or less of the cells in the tumor are normal. These cells do not resemble any family member. Usually most aggressive.

Scarff/Bloom/Richardson Tumor Grading Scale

Some pathologists use the **Scarff/Bloom/Richardson** grading scale. This grading system gives a number from 1 to 3 according to aggressiveness of three different characteristics: 1- tubular formation, 2- nuclear size and shape, 3 - mitotic count. The numbers from each characteristic are then totaled to determine the aggressiveness of a tumor. The higher the number, the more aggressive are the characteristics of the tumor.

Characteristics Evaluated Using the Scarff/Bloom/Richardson Grading Scale:

Evaluates cell arrangements for characteristics of looking like a small tube.

1. Tubular Formation	Grade Value
Majority >75%	1
Moderate degree 10 - 75%	2
Little or none	3

Evaluates size and shape variation of cells and nucleus of cells.

2. Nuclear Shape/Size	Grade Value
Uniform nuclear shapes	1
Moderate increase in varying shapes	2
Marked variation (often large nucleus)	3

Determines how many cells are visible in the dividing stage in an area of the tumor.

3. Cell Division Rate	Grade Value
Low (0 - 5)	1
Moderate (6 - 10)	2
High (>11)	3

Total of the scores in the above three areas of evaluation determines final grade.

Final Cumulative Total	Points
Grade 1 - well differentiated	3 - 5 points
Grade 2 - moderately differentiated	6 - 7 points
Grade 3 - poorly differentiated	8 - 9 points

A higher final Scarff/Bloom/Richardson score indicates a more aggressive tumor.

Prognostic Indicators Other Than Grade

♦ **Necrosis** (cell death) may be noted in a report. Cell death is a result of the lack of necessary oxygen and nutrients to parts of a tumor causing the cell to die. This signifies a more aggressive cancer. Often necrosis is related to a comedo (type of aggressive cell) component.

♦ **Blood Vessel (Vascular) or Lymphatic Invasion**
A microscopic examination of the tumor will show if the surrounding blood vessels or lymphatic vessels have been invaded by the tumor. No invasion offers a better prognosis.

Prognostic Tests

Various tests may be ordered to look at specific characteristics of the tumor cells.
♦ **DNA Status:**
A test that looks at the genetic material found in the DNA (blueprint for cell reproduction) of a cell. Normal DNA of a cell appears with two sets of chromosomes.
DNA ploidy determines DNA composition of cells. Tumors may be:
• **Diploid** means having two sets of chromosomes, which is normal.
• **Aneuploid** refers to the characteristic of having either fewer than or more than two sets of chromosomes; this is abnormal, suggesting aggression.
DNA index is the ratio of aneuploid DNA compared to diploid DNA.

64

Proliferation Markers

◆ **S Phase Fraction** – Flow cytometry reveals number of dividing cells and corresponds to the growth rate of a tumor.

◆ **Mitotic Rate** – Microscopic observation of number of cells that are dividing.

◆ **Ki67 Stain** – Microscopic observation of all dividing cells.

Increase in any of the above proliferation markers suggests an aggressive tumor.

Hormone Receptor Assay

A hormone receptor assay is a chemical or observation test that measures the presence of **estrogen** and **progesterone receptors** in the tumor cells. It tells the physician whether the tumor was stimulated to grow by female hormones and is very important in determining what type of treatment will be used. If a tumor is positive, that means it was stimulated by estrogen or progesterone and usually carries a slight increase in a positive prognosis. Positive receptor tumors may be treated with anti-hormonal medications (Tamoxifen) for control.

Tumors may be:
ER+ (positive) and PR+ (positive)
ER- (negative) and PR+ (positive)
ER+ (positive) and PR- (negative)
ER- (negative) and PR- (negative).

HER-2/neu (c-erbB-2) Oncogene (substances in cells that promote tumor development)

This oncogene is found amplified and over-expressed in about 20-30% of breast cancers. Recently it has been demonstrated that HER-2/neu over-expression can predict the response to Adriamycin-based chemotherapy, as well as resistance to Tamoxifen. Furthermore, the recent introduction of immunotherapy with a "humanized" monoclonal antibody, Transmuxtab (Herceptin™) directed at the HER-2/neu protein, has required further screening of breast cancers for HER-2/neu over-expression to determine if these types of drugs may be effective.

There are many other diagnostic tests being used to evaluate tumors. Your physician will discuss with you the tests selected to evaluate your tumor. Each of these tests helps collect pieces of the puzzle needed for the oncologist to determine your best treatment.

The pathologist prepares a written report that is sent to your physician. Time varies as to when the final report will be available. Check with your physician on how long your laboratory requires. After reviewing the pathology report, your physician will decide if further diagnostic tests, such as a bone scan, liver scan, chest x-ray, CT scan or an MRI (magnetic resonance imager), may be needed to stage your cancer.

Staging of Cancer

When all test results are complete, your cancer will be staged on a scale from **zero (in-situ cancer) to stage four (a cancer with distant metastasis)**. A stage zero cancer is the least aggressive with the best prognosis. Staging is an estimate of how much the cancer has spread and is important in the selection of appropriate treatment. The three basic factors considered in staging are: 1- tumor size, 2 - lymph node involvement, 3- metastasis to other areas of the body.

Stage 0: Tumor in situ; negative nodes

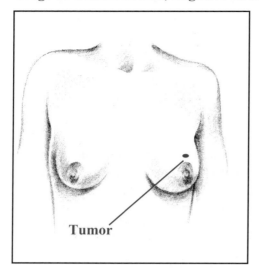

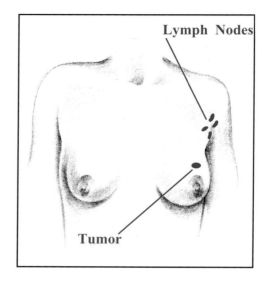

Stage I: Tumor confined to breast, 2 cm or smaller; negative nodes

Stage II: Tumor 2-5 cm; movable positive axillary nodes; or tumor over 5 cm with negative nodes

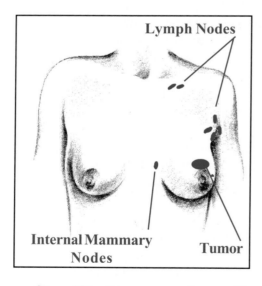

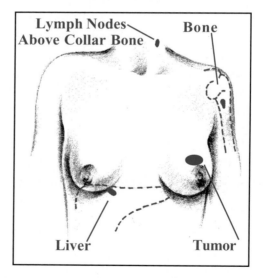

Stage III: Tumor over 5 cm with positive nodes; or involvement of skin, fixed axillary nodes or internal mammary nodes

Stage IV: Distant Metastasis

When you return to the physician for your pathology results, you may want to ask the following questions and write down the answers. Some doctors will provide a copy of your pathology report for your records, and some pathologists will be happy to talk to you.

Questions To Ask About Your Pathology Report
- What is the name of the type of cancer I have?
- Was my tumor in situ (inside ducts or lobules) or infiltrating (invasive--grown through the duct or lobule walls)?
- What size was my tumor? (The size is in centimeters (cm) or millimeters (mm). 10 mm equals 1 cm. 1 cm equals 3/8 inch. 1 inch equals approximately 2.5 cm.)
- Was the cancer found anywhere else in my breast tissue? (Multifocal means found in the same quadrant as the tumor. Multicentric is in another quadrant of the breast.)
- How many lymph nodes were removed? How many levels of lymph nodes did you sample or remove? (You have three levels of nodes.)
- Were any nodes positive with cancer cells?
- Were my tumor receptors estrogen or progesterone positive or negative? Was the tumor HER-2/neu positive or negative?
- Was my cancer diploid (like a normal, original cell) or aneuploid?
- How fast was my cancer growing? (S phase or mitotic index)
- Is there anything else that I need to know about my cancer?

After the Pathology Report

As a patient you do not have any control over what your pathology report contains. However, as an educated, informed patient, you can join forces with your physicians in defeating the disease.

Chemotherapy

Chemotherapy comes from two words which mean chemical and treatment. We have all experienced treatment with chemicals for other illnesses, such as antibiotics for infections and cold medicines. The word **chemotherapy** is usually a term that refers to treatment for cancer through the use of drugs. After surgery for cancer, treatment with chemotherapy, hormonal therapy or radiation therapy is often referred to as **adjuvant** (additional) **therapy.** Adjuvant therapy is given to prevent a recurrence of cancer by killing any undetected cells that may remain in your body. Sometimes several doses of chemotherapy may be given **before** surgery to shrink a tumor, called **neoadjuvant chemotherapy.** If a tumor shrinks, this serves as a barometer of how well the selected drugs will work at killing remaining cancerous cells in the body after surgery. Adjuvant chemotherapy is then given after surgery is completed. Your physicians will determine which one or combination of adjuvant therapies you may require.

How Does Chemotherapy Work?

Chemotherapy works by killing cells that are dividing in your body. The cancer cells are constantly dividing until something disrupts this cycle. This disruption is the role of chemotherapy. Even when the surgeon feels all of your tumor has been removed, you may receive adjuvant chemotherapy because there is a possibility that some cells may have broken away from the original site and moved through the lymphatic or blood vessels to other parts of your body **(metastasis)** where they cannot be detected; this is called **micrometastasis** (too small to be detected). Adjuvant chemotherapy helps destroy these cells. Chemotherapy and hormonal therapy are effective in all parts of the body, whereas radiation therapy treats only the breast.

Because chemotherapy works by killing dividing cells, most of the side effects will be on the cells in your body that are constantly dividing to produce new cells. These cells are found in your bone marrow, where your blood components are made, resulting in lowered blood cell counts; in the gastrointestinal tract, resulting in a possible sore throat or mouth; and in hair follicles, which could result in hair loss. Most of these cells are able to recover quickly when treatment is over. Therefore, these side effects are over quickly. Some people experience very few side effects and are able to continue to work throughout treatment.

Don't listen to anyone else and their stories about the side effects of chemotherapy. Instead, ask your nurse for the name of the drugs prescribed for you and the side effects for those particular drugs. There are currently about 50 drugs being used to treat cancer, and there are about 100 types of cancer which include approximately 15 different types of breast cancer. Therefore, it would be difficult to get accurate information from anyone but medical professionals involved with cancer treatment.

Your First Oncologist's Visit

It is very important when planning your first visit to the oncologist to carry a list of any medications that you take. Include nonprescription medicines such as cold or sinus pills, aspirin, antacids, laxatives and vitamins or herbs as well. Many drugs can alter the response of the treatment, and your oncologist will need to evaluate if you can continue the medication. Check with your oncologist before starting any new medication.

Your oncologist will carefully review your pathology report and any other tests, perform a thorough physical exam and then prescribe a treatment plan. This treatment plan will be designed according to:

◆ cancer cell type

◆ size of tumor

◆ in situ or invasive cancer

◆ growth rate of tumor

◆ evidence of spread of cancer to other parts of the body

◆ lymph node involvement

◆ how much the cells have changed from original cells

◆ estrogen and progesterone hormone receptor status

◆ your menopausal state

◆ your medical history

◆ your general health

Remember, there is more than one kind of breast cancer, and different types of cancers may require different treatments. Some types of cancer, or cancer that has spread to other parts of the body, **may** require chemotherapy administration **before surgery** is performed. **Do not compare your treatment with another patient's treatment**, because you will probably be comparing two completely different cases. Also, information you read in the paper or magazines or reports on radio or television may not be applicable to your cancer. Rely on your physician and staff to be assured you are receiving accurate information relevant to your treatment.

Chemotherapy Drug Selection

A combination of several drugs may be used to fight your cancer. The drugs selected will have different side effects and work in different ways to kill the cancer cells. They are used to attack any cancer cells that may be left in the body at different phases of the cell division. Your doctor may also add an anti-hormonal drug, **Tamoxifen**, that you will take by mouth. Anti-hormonal drugs are drugs that block the hormone receptors on breast tissue and cause very few side effects. **Immunotherapy** treatments, which stimulate your immune system in specific ways that allow your own body to fight the cancer, may also be used.

How Chemotherapy Is Given

Chemotherapy drugs may be given by mouth, as an injection into the muscle or fatty tissues or into a vein by an I.V. (intravenous) needle. If your veins are hard to locate or you are to receive certain types of chemotherapy drugs, some doctors may request the insertion of a permanent I.V. site (referred to as a vascular access device, a port—"life port" or "port-a-cath"). This is a device inserted by a surgeon under the skin, usually on the chest opposite your surgery site and occasionally on the arm. This device may be used to draw your blood for blood studies as well as to administer chemotherapy and other medications. It prevents repeated needle sticks to your arm. You are able to bathe and swim as usual with a port.

Chemotherapy may be administered in the doctor's office, a hospital or in a clinic. Most breast cancer patients take treatments in a physician's office or clinic. Some chemotherapy, however, may be administered by wearing an infusion pump (which is the size of a transistor radio and runs on batteries). An infusion pump allows continuous, around-the-clock delivery of the chemotherapy for several days at a time at home.

Chemotherapy Scheduling

The frequency of treatments may vary, just as doses will vary from patient to patient. It will depend on the kind of cancer, the drugs being used and how your body responds to them. Some drugs are given by mouth daily. Others may be scheduled biweekly, weekly, every three weeks or by other schedules. Most breast cancer chemotherapy by vein is on a three to four week schedule in a physician's office or clinic. Your oncologist will be able to tell you about a treatment plan and schedule after your case has been evaluated. This schedule may be readjusted to meet your individual response and treatment needs. Treatments are usually begun after surgery; however, some types of cancer require chemotherapy administration before surgery.

Chemotherapy Side Effects

You have probably heard horrible stories about cancer treatments. Times have changed. There are new drugs that have changed many treatment side effects. A new drug for nausea has greatly reduced vomiting as a side effect. Drugs can now be given to elevate your immune response during treatment, preventing many of the infections traditionally experienced. Ask your nurse and doctor to tell you about the side effects of your treatment plan. Do not rely on well-meaning friends or family. Chemotherapy has been repeatedly successful in increasing survival from breast cancer. (See Appendix B for types of drugs.)

Hormonal Therapy

Hormonal therapy may be recommended by your oncologist. This type of additional anti-cancer therapy is prescribed after surgery for some women if their cancer pathology report revealed the tumor was dependent on the female hormones, estrogen or progesterone, to grow. Tumors that have a significant number of estrogen receptors (ER) are considered "ER positive," and tumors that have a high number of progesterone receptors are considered "PR positive." Receptor status of the tumor determines what treatments will best affect your cancer. Use of hormonal drugs often depends upon whether you are pre-menopausal (having your monthly menstrual periods) or post-menopausal (not having your monthly menstrual periods).

Tamoxifen Citrate

The most widely used drug to alter the hormonal stimulation of the breast after breast cancer is Tamoxifen citrate (Nolvadex®). While most doctors are not exactly sure how Tamoxifen works, most acknowledge that it prevents breast cancer cells from getting the estrogen they need to grow. When the drug is released into the bloodstream, the molecules attach to the estrogen receptors on the cancer cells and prevent or slow their growth but do not kill the cancer cells. Chemotherapy drugs work by destroying cells, including healthy cells in the blood, scalp, mouth and gastrointestinal tract. Tamoxifen does **not** destroy healthy cells in your body. Side effects experienced with chemotherapy are **not** experienced with anti-hormonal therapy. Some women report an increased sense of well-being after taking the drug because of its estrogen-like effects on other organs of the body. Tamoxifen has been proven to protect a woman against heart disease and osteoporosis.

Tamoxifen is taken by pill, usually twice a day. The most frequently reported side effects of Tamoxifen occur when the drug is started. Some women may have mild nausea that subsides shortly. If the drug is taken with food, nausea is less likely to occur. Hot flashes are also reported. For most women, these side effects are easily tolerated. Your physician will tell you if you are a candidate for hormonal therapy.

Autologous Stem Cell Transplant

A new aggressive treatment for breast cancer is available in some treatment centers, autologous (taken from your own body) stem cell (immature, parent blood cell) transplant. This procedure may be recommended if the cancer has spread outside of the breast to other areas of the body. Numerous guidelines and criteria regarding age, extent of disease and prior treatment are factors that are considered for the recommendation of stem cell therapy.

The autologous stem cell process begins with the administration of several doses of chemotherapy into a vein. Drugs are then given to promote the development of stem cells in the blood. The stem cells are collected from the blood through a process call leukapheresis (removal of white blood cells containing stem cells). The removed cells are stored for future return to the body. Large doses of chemotherapy are then given to the patient over a period of three to five days to aggressively attack remaining cancer cells in the body. The patient's own stored stem cells are returned to the body several days later through an I.V. infusion, much like a blood transfusion, to rescue the body from the effects of the large doses of chemotherapy. Ten days to several weeks of hospitalization are required after the infusion to monitor for potential infection and the body's response to the treatment.

Bone Marrow Transplant

A very aggressive treatment for breast cancer is bone marrow transplant. The procedure is performed in a medical center specializing in bone marrow transplantation. Guidelines to qualify vary at different centers, but usually factors considered are: disease outside of the breast tissue, your age and your general health status. This procedure may or may not be covered by insurance.

Aggressive large dose chemotherapy, with the goal of eradicating all cancer cells at once, can severely limit the bone marrow function of the body, necessitating having marrow for replacement. Therefore, bone marrow is removed from the body (**autologous**, from own body) by inserting large bore needles into the large bones of the body, often the bones in the hip area, and **aspirating** (pulling back into a large syringe) the cells that form the blood components. The removed marrow is stored for later use. After large doses of chemotherapy are given, the autologous bone marrow is returned to the body through an I.V. needle, much like a blood transfusion. The treatment is relatively new for breast cancer patients, and there are many side effects that may be experienced during and after treatment. Your physician may discuss this treatment option if your cancer requires aggressive treatment.

Questions You May Wish to Ask an Oncologist

- What kind of treatment will I receive (chemotherapy, hormonal)?
- On what schedule will I receive these treatments?
- How long will I receive treatments?
- Where will I receive my treatments (office, clinic, hospital)?
- Can someone come with me to receive my treatments?
- How long will each treatment take?
- Will I feel like driving myself home after my treatment, or do I need a driver?
- What are the names of the drugs I will receive?
- Are they given by mouth or in a vein?
- Will I need a port (device implanted under the skin) to receive any I.V. medications, or will you use a vein in my arm?

◆ What side effects will I experience from the treatments (nausea, hair loss, changes in blood cell counts, etc.)?

◆ Will I be given medications to treat side effects?

◆ Should I eat before I come for my treatments?

◆ Do I continue to take previous medications during these treatments?

◆ Can I take vitamins or herbs if I so choose?

◆ What kind of protective precautions to my skin should I take during chemotherapy (against exposure to sunlight)?

◆ Will any other tests be given before or while I receive my chemotherapy?

◆ Will I continue to have my menstrual periods? If not, when will they return?

◆ Should I use birth control? What type do you recommend?

◆ Will I be able to conceive and bear a child after treatments?

◆ What physical changes should I report to you or to your nurse during treatment?

◆ Will I need radiation therapy?

◆ Can I continue my usual work or exercise schedule during treatments?

◆ Are there any precautions my family should take to limit exposure to the chemotherapy during my treatments (shared eating utensils, bathroom facilities)?

◆ How will you evaluate the effectiveness of the treatments?

◆ When I complete my treatments how often will I return for checkups?

◆ Do you have written information on my cancer or treatment plans?

Radiation Therapy

A **radiation oncologist** is a physician who specializes in using radiation (x-ray) therapy to treat diseases. If your physician feels that radiation therapy could kill any remaining cancer cells in your breast, you will be referred to a radiation oncologist for evaluation. After reviewing your pathology report, all diagnostic test findings and surgery report, the radiation oncologist will perform a physical exam and write a prescription for the dosage of radiation and the exact area to be treated.

Understanding Radiation Therapy

Radiation therapy is delivered by a machine that produces high-energy x-rays from radioactive substances. The radiation is directed to the area in your body where diagnostic reports identified disease or potential for microscopic disease. The series of treatments has the ability to kill remaining cells in the treated area. This energy is like that used in x-rays, only stronger. It is painless, and you cannot see the rays. Because radiation therapy lessens the size of the tumor mass and alleviates tumor pressure, it can also be used for cancer pain control.

Lumpectomy is usually followed with radiation therapy to the breast area for five to six weeks.

First Radiation Therapy Visit

On your first visit you will go through a process to calculate the exact area to be radiated. X-ray pictures or a CAT scan may be taken to determine precisely where to direct the rays of radiation. These areas will be marked carefully on your body to assure that your treatment is delivered to the exact place it is needed.

Receiving Radiation Therapy Treatments

Treatments are given as an outpatient on a daily basis Monday through Friday. Even though the actual radiation therapy takes only a few minutes to deliver, it may take 15 to 30 minutes to prepare the room and the equipment. When you receive your treatment, you will lie on your back on a table in a room with your arm placed above your head. You may have a special form or pad placed to help you maintain your position. You will be alone but monitored by a camera outside of the treatment room with the ability to talk to the technician over an intercom.

Side Effects of Treatment

Throughout the therapy your radiation oncologist will check on the effects of the treatments. The side effects from the radiation are mild. Some experience mild fatigue, slight skin discoloration in the area(resembling a sunburn), sore throat, difficulty swallowing or a dry cough. Radiation treatments are painless during delivery, do not make you radioactive, nor do they make you a danger to your family.

Questions You May Wish to Ask a Radiation Oncologist

- How many radiation treatments will I receive?
- How long will my first visit take to mark the area?
- How do you mark the area that will be radiated?
- What kind of soap and bath do you recommend during the treatments?
- Is there anything that I cannot use during my treatment (deodorant, perfume, lotions to the chest or back, etc.)?
- Can I wear a bra or my prosthesis?
- Do you have written information on radiation therapy for the breast area?
- What side effects are considered normal during therapy?
- What side effects, if they occur, should I report immediately?

ॐ ॐ ॐ

> Refer to the tear-out worksheets, "Oncologist's Questions" and "Radiation Oncologist's Questions," at the back of the book.

*As Survivors,
we go beyond brokenness and
overcome tragedy and hurts because
we do things differently during our
grief and healing process. We
know that what we think and what
we do can make a difference in our
recovery. Therefore, we measure
carefully our thoughts and actions to
keep them positive, making this part
of our treatment plan
for recovery.*

Chapter 10

Monitoring Your Physical Recovery

"I give a great deal of credit to my Reach to Recovery visitor for my physical recovery. She provided me with a wealth of information. For the first time, I had something I could read and re-read. I was discovering fast the necessity of education in this new and strange world."

~ Harriett Barrineau, survivor

After surgery for breast cancer, there are areas of your health that you will monitor. You will need to exercise your surgical arm for return of range of motion and learn how to prevent or treat lymphedema. Breast self-exam on the remaining breast(s) and the incision site, along with mammograms and clinical exams by a physician, will help you monitor for any potential recurrence. Dietary habits and physical exercise may help your recovery and add to your physical well-being. These are areas you can take responsibility for monitoring.

Surgical Arm Changes

After your surgery, the area of your incision will have diminished sensation, and your arm may feel numb or tingly. The area under the arm, where the lymph nodes are removed, contains nerves that, if injured or cut, can cause different types of sensations. The most common is numbness or a tingling sensation. The area under your arm and the back of your arm is where the numbness usually occurs. If the nerve is stretched or injured during surgery, there can be numbness or a tingling sensation which may improve in a few months. If the nerve is cut, the numbness will be permanent. However, this will not affect the use of your arm.

The surgical arm will feel very tight when you attempt to stretch it out over your head. Removing your lymph nodes also required the removal of an area of fat with the lymph nodes. This causes the area to feel pulled and tight after surgery. This is temporary and will improve as you begin your exercise program and gradually stretch this area.

After surgery, your surgical arm needs to be exercised to restore normal range of motion. (The "surgical arm" is the arm on the side of your surgery, and the "non-surgical arm" is the opposite arm.) **However, do not begin any exercises until your surgeon gives you permission.** Most physicians prefer that all drains, sutures or staples be removed before attempting an exercise routine. Ask your physician when to begin range of motion exercises. Additional instructions as to types of exercises may be provided by your physician.

Your Arm Exercise Program

When you begin the exercise program, you will find that you may tire easily and that there will be some discomfort as you attempt to perform the movements. However, continue to perform them to the point of slight discomfort but **not until it becomes painful.** It may take several weeks before you are able to complete some of the exercises. Work at your own pace. Your progress will be gradual. Some women find that by taking their pain medication, aspirin, Advil® or Tylenol® an hour before starting, or by taking a warm shower just prior to beginning the exercises, the routine is less uncomfortable.

Exercises should be performed on a **regular basis, preferably two or more sessions a day, 10 to 15 minutes each session**. Persistence is the key to regaining complete range of motion. Do the exercises slowly and hold the position when you get to the end of the range. This helps stretch and strengthen the muscles. Some exercises require a small rubber ball to squeeze and a broom handle or yardstick to hold in your hand. Many of the exercises may be performed either standing or sitting down.

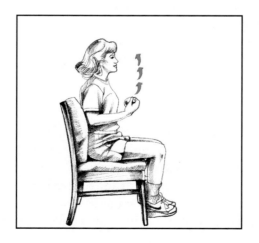 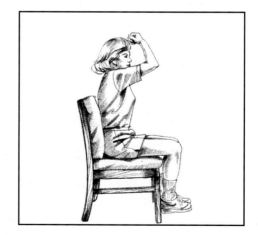

Surgical Arm Raises

Clench a rubber ball in your surgical hand with your elbow bent. Slowly lift your arm toward your head. Keep your elbow away from your body as you lift the ball toward your head. Hold your position for a few seconds when you reach your head. Repeat six times.

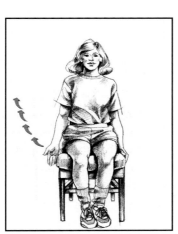
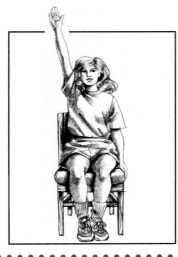

Surgical Arm Lifts

Lift your surgical arm away from your side toward the ceiling with your palm turned forward. Raise your arm as high as possible and hold it there for a few seconds. Repeat six times.

Surgical Arm Reach

Hold your surgical arm straight beside your body. Slowly raise your arm as high as possible over your head while keeping your elbow straight. Hold the position for a few seconds. Repeat six times.

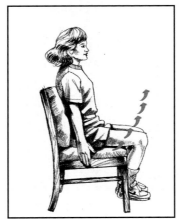
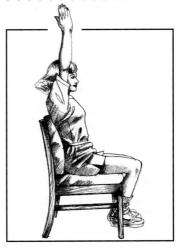

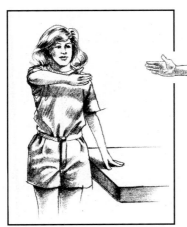
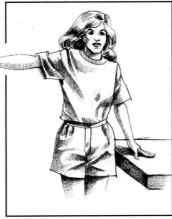

Surgical Arm Swings

Place your non-surgical arm on a table to support your body. Put your surgical arm across your chest, placing your hand on the opposite shoulder. Move the surgical arm slowly away from your body until it is extended straight out. Keep your arm at shoulder level as you perform the exercise. Repeat six times.

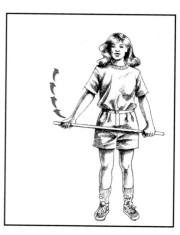
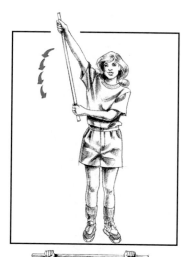

Range of Motion

Hold a stick with your surgical hand palm up and your non-surgical arm palm down, as you push your surgical arm directly out from your side toward the ceiling until you feel a stretch. Hold this position for several seconds. Repeat six times.

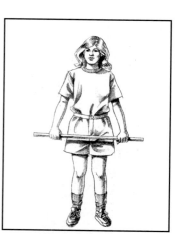
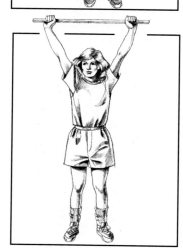

Bring the stick directly over your head, leading with the non-surgical arm. Reach back over your head until you feel a stretch. Hold the position for a few seconds and repeat six times.

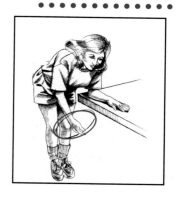
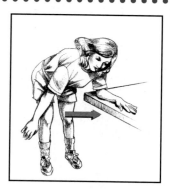
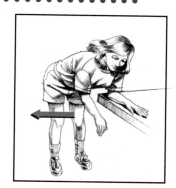

Surgical Arm Circles and Arm Swings

Lean on a table with your non-surgical arm. Move your surgical arm in a circle clockwise and then counterclockwise. Repeat six times. Leaning on the table, as before, swing your surgical arm from side to side six times.

If you are having difficulty performing the exercises and feel you are not making progress, tell your surgeon. Some women need the assistance of a physical therapist to regain complete range of motion, or they may need the motivation of an exercise group led by a professional.

After breast surgery, it is not uncommon for some women to favor the use of their non-surgical arm and become "one armed" as they resume their daily activities. Weakness in the surgical arm, which most women experience to some degree, will cause this to happen. However, it is helpful if you remember that using the surgical arm normally will gradually increase strength and range of motion.

Lymphedema Prevention and Management

Removal of the lymph nodes under your surgical arm or radiation therapy to the underarm area may cause a swelling called **lymphedema**. (**Lymph,** from lymphatic fluid; **edema,** swelling from fluid accumulation.) This condition results in swelling from the slower flow and removal of lymphatic fluid from your arm. Only a small percentage of women experience lymphedema after healing from surgery, but all women need to know of the potential and treatment if it should occur. It can occur anytime from shortly after surgery to years later.

Arm lymphedema can produce pain, restricted movement of the shoulder and arm and increased susceptibility to infection. Medications and treatments are often limited in their effectiveness; therefore, the best strategy is to **prevent** the problem before it occurs.

Lymphedema may be related to:
- infection
- poor range of motion in your surgical arm
- obesity
- radiation therapy to the breast and underarm area
- constriction caused by clothing or jewelry
- long periods of positioning the arm below the level of the heart
- repetitious task using the surgical arm

The first line of defense against lymphedema is regaining full range of motion of your arm by using the exercises suggested in this book or by your physician. While these exercises may seem dull and unnecessary, they serve to facilitate the flow of the lymphatic fluid from the arm area. **Do not begin an exercise program until your physician gives you permission.**

Steps to Help Prevent Arm Lymphedema

- For several weeks after surgery, when lying down, prop your arm up on a pillow above the level of your heart to help drain the fluid. Elevation of the arm helps reduce swelling and prevents additional accumulation of fluid.

- Keep your arm slightly out from your body, so as not to compress the underarm area. Using a small pillow or a small stuffed animal under your arm when sitting will keep the arm away from the body and keep swelling at a minimum. Some swelling under the arm is expected due to surgery and will improve with time.

- Avoid using your arm and hand in a dependent position (below the level of the heart) for long periods of time. If you need to perform a task of this sort, periodically hold your arms above your head to promote drainage.

- Make a fist or squeeze a small rubber ball in your hand repetitively for two to three minutes several times a day to assist the accumulated fluid in returning to general circulation.

Steps to Avoid Injury and Infection

- Do not allow the surgical arm to be used for blood pressure checks, blood samples or injections. Ask your nurse for a pink wristband or ribbon to be placed on the wrist of your surgical arm as a reminder to all your health care givers.

- Do not wear anything that is tight on the arm or hand, such as rings, watches, bracelets or tight elastic in sleeves.

- Do not hold a cigarette in this hand.

- Do not cut your cuticles; keep hands soft by using hand lotion regularly.

- Do not carry heavy packages or purses on the side of your surgery.

- Wear protective gloves when working in the garden, washing dishes or using any irritating chemicals, such as hair dye or cleaning products.

- Avoid burns and cuts when cooking.

- Wash all cuts or injuries with antibacterial soap, apply an antibacterial medication, and cover the area with sterile gauze or a Band-Aid® until the wound heals.

- Avoid sunburn. Wear long sleeves or a sunscreen at all times when in direct sunlight for a period of time.

◆ Use a thimble when sewing.

◆ Avoid insect bites by wearing insect repellent.

◆ Be careful with animals. Avoid scratches.

◆ Use an electric razor under your arm.

When To Notify Your Physician

These precautions may help you to avoid injury and a potential for infection in your arm. If you ever experience any **redness**, **pain** or **infection** in this arm or hand, notify your physician. If you injure the arm or hand and run a low-grade **fever, contact your doctor.** When accumulated lymph fluid becomes infected with bacteria and inflames the surrounding tissue, it is a condition called **cellulitis.** Antibiotics will be necessary to treat the infection. Early intervention is necessary to prevent the spread of infection to other parts of your body.

Treatment For Lymphedema In the Surgical Arm

If you have persistent swelling several weeks after your surgery, the first treatment is simply to elevate the arm. Raising the arm above the level of the heart by propping it on a pillow for 45 minutes several times a day will usually reduce most lymphedema. Sleeping with the arm elevated on a pillow is helpful. If the swelling persists after elevation, notify your physician.

A special hand massage method, **Manual Lymph Drainage (MLD),** is taught by some physical therapists or massage therapists. Patients and family members are instructed to use their hands in stroking movements, using pressure to remove lymph fluid from the arm. Your physician may recommend a physical or massage therapist with these skills. Steps to manage swelling in the arm should begin when you first notice it occurring.

A special elastic sleeve (Jobst sleeve) designed to reduce swelling may be ordered by the physician. The sleeve looks much like a support hose and can be worn under long-sleeved clothing. A professional fitter will measure the arm and make a customized sleeve to fit your measurements. If the swelling continues, a special sleeve hooked to a compression pump may be used several hours a day to manually remove the accumulated fluid. Both the sleeve and the compression pump must be ordered by a physician.

Remember, lymphedema usually has **nothing to do with cancer**. This condition occurs because lymph nodes and vessels in the breast have been removed during surgery; scar tissue has formed after surgery or radiation therapy has caused changes in the area. These conditions slow down the removal of the lymphatic fluid that accumulates in the breast and arm area, resulting in swelling of the arm and hand.

Assessing Range of Motion

After having performed your exercises for several months following your surgery, ask the following questions to determine whether you have adequate return of motion in your arm.

If you could perform the following prior to surgery, can you now easily:

- Brush and comb your hair?

- Pull a tee shirt or tight-necked sweater over your head?

- Close a back-fastening bra?

- Completely zip up a dress that has a back-long zipper?

- Wash the upper part of your back in the shoulder blade area of the opposite side of surgery?

- Reach over your head into a cabinet to remove an object?

- Make a double bed?

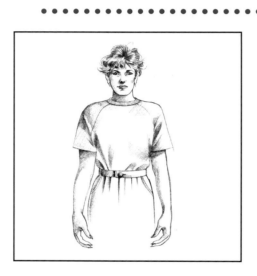 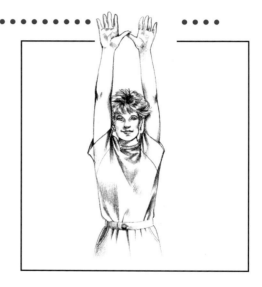

Full Range of Motion Exercise

With both of your arms straight by your side, raise both hands above your head and hold the position for several seconds. Repeat six times. This exercise will be one of the last to master and will be proof that your surgical arm has regained full range of motion.

When you can master this exercise, congratulate yourself on the hard work required to stick with your dull, routine exercise program to accomplish this task. If you have not regained your range of motion, talk with your surgeon about a physical therapist or an exercise program led by a professional trained in range of motion exercises.

Remember

- Exercise is essential to restore normal use of your surgical arm.

- Exercise to the point of some discomfort but not pain.

ॐ Protect your surgical arm from injury.

ॐ Treat lymphedema by elevating your surgical arm. If this is not successful, call your physician.

ॐ Immediately report any sign of infection in your surgical arm .

Breast Self-Exam After Surgery

Much time will be spent the first year seeing physicians regarding your surgeries and treatments. During this time they will be monitoring many areas of your health. However, there are several areas of your health that you will need to oversee. One of these is the monthly breast self-exam (BSE) on the remaining breast and the mastectomy scar area or the scar area of the lumpectomy breast.

Many women state it is difficult for them to perform BSE after having cancer. It is helpful if you can master this fear. Early detection is your surest weapon against breast cancer. There is a small possibility that you could develop cancer in the other breast or have a recurrence in the remaining breast tissue in a lumpectomy breast or scar area of a mastectomy. To keep a vigilant guard on your health, you need to check your breast(s) on a regular basis and report any suspicious changes to your physician. It is important to remember that women find most of the suspicious lumps and that finding them early greatly increases the chances for a successful treatment.

Some women have found it helpful to have a physician examine their breast(s) and explain what they feel and assure them that everything in the breast(s) at this time is a normal finding. This exam gives the assurance needed to start their own program of regular examinations, knowing that the breasts have no known abnormalities.

When to Start Your Breast Self-Exam After Surgery

◆ Lumpectomy patients should begin breast self-exam at the completion of radiation therapy or when the incision has healed completely.

◆ Mastectomy patients should begin examination of the surgical site approximately two to three months after surgery. You should carefully examine the scar and surrounding area.

◆ Reconstructive surgery patients should examine the entire reconstruction area beginning when their incision is completely healed, approximately two to three months after the surgery.

When to Perform Your Monthly Exam

It is recommended that all women perform breast self-exams once a month. Select a quiet, uninterrupted time when you can concentrate. A breast self-exam is especially important since you have had breast cancer.

- ◆ **Menstruating women** should check their breast(s) the last day of the menstrual period or several days past.
- ◆ **Post-menopausal women** should check their breast(s) the same day of each month.
- ◆ **Women receiving treatment** who are not having a regular menstrual period need to select the same day each month.

How To Learn What Is Normal After Surgery

Your goal in breast self-exam is to carefully check your breast(s) to learn what is normal for you. All women's breasts feel differently because of the differences in body tissue and the stimulation of their body hormones on these tissues. Lumpiness in the breast often results because of hormonal changes in the tissues. This is referred to as **normal nodularity**. After checking your breast(s) regularly, you will discover a normal nodularity pattern in your breast(s). Your goal will then be to check for distinct changes in your breast(s), especially new lumps, and report these changes to your doctor.

Pain in a surgical breast which is sporadic, with a shooting sensation, is not uncommon in the incision area, especially in breast conserving surgery. This pain can occur for months.

Incision scars may have areas that feel firm to touch, which is caused by scar tissue formation during healing. Areas where drains were inserted may also feel firm. You will need to become familiar with these changes soon after your surgery. This will prevent misinterpretation of these normal post-surgical changes. Very rarely does cancer recur in the incisional area the first months after surgery. Your physician can help you distinguish and identify these changes.

Changes In The Radiated Breast

The radiated breast may experience the following changes:
- ◆ Darkening in color of the area (suntanned appearance)
- ◆ Edema (swelling) of the breast tissues for up to a year
- ◆ Gradual decrease in swelling
- ◆ A firmness of the radiated tissues, often feeling lumpy to touch
- ◆ Skin thickening, greatest in the area of the nipple and areola in breast conserving surgery
- ◆ Slight decrease in size of the radiated breast when edema subsides
- ◆ Decreased sensitivity of the breast

It is helpful to become familiar with the normal changes occurring after radiation. Some women feel that applying powder or hand lotion to their hands prior to their self-exam assists in moving their hands freely over the breast tissue.

The exam described below has been taken from the **MammaCare®** method. This method was developed from research at the University of Florida and is now considered state-of-the-art in breast self-exam techniques. Components of the MammaCare® exam are as follows:

Position for Exam

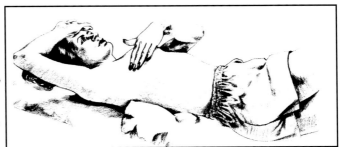

- Lie down on a bed on the side opposite of the breast you will examine.
- Pull your knees up slightly, rotate the shoulder (of the breast you will examine) to the flat of the bed.

(You may place a small pillow under the arch of the back to increase comfort.)

- Place your hand **palm up** on your **forehead**.
- Use your right hand to examine your left breast and your left hand to examine your right breast, reaching across your body.
- Remain in the side-lying position until you reach the nipple, then roll **flat on your back and place your arm by your side** to continue your exam.

The side-lying position, for a portion of the exam, allows a woman, especially one with large breast(s), to most effectively examine the outer half of the breast by spreading out the tissues evenly. Fifty percent of all cancers occur in the quarter of the breast that extends from the nipple to underneath the arm. When a woman lies flat on her back the breast tissue naturally falls into this area. The side-lying position prevents this from occurring. When you reach the nipple and turn to your back, you cause the inner half of the breast to be spread out as thin as possible for your exam.

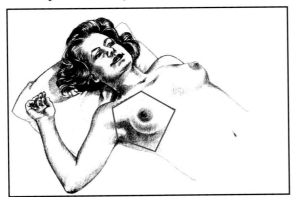

Area To Be Examined

The area to be examined is from the middle notch in your collarbone, following under collarbone until you reach mid-underarm, straight down until you reach your bra line. Follow bra line to middle of breastbone and back to notch.

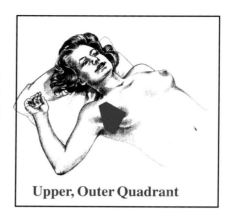

The reason for the new larger boundaries is that the breast is a large gland that covers most of this area, not just the breast mound. Remember that 50 percent of cancers occur in the upper, outer quadrant of the breast. Examine this area carefully.

Upper, Outer Quadrant

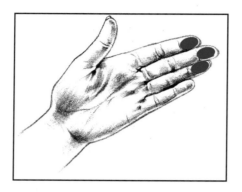

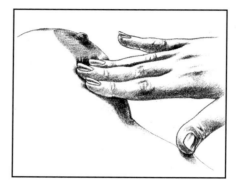

Finger Positions

Use the flats of **three** middle fingers, the first joint down to tips. Place flats of fingers in a flat bowing position on the breast tissue.

Pressures

Three levels of pressure will be used when making circles.

◆ **Light pressure**—barely moves the top layer of skin.

◆ **Medium pressure**—goes halfway through the thickness of breast tissue.

◆ **Deep pressure**—goes to the base of the breast next to ribs.

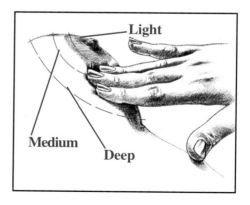

Use varying pressures so you can examine carefully the full thickness of the breast, without displacing small lumps into fibrous tissue or your rib area. Pressures do not injure your breast tissue. **Do not lift your hand or release the pressure** as you make these three circles.

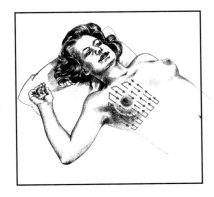

Pattern of Search

Begin under your arm and make rows of straight lines up and down on the breast tissue, just as if you were mowing your grass. Ten to 16 vertical strips will be needed.

Using the MammaCare® Components to Examine Your Breast(s)

◆ Assume the side-lying position with your hand on your forehead, **palm up** and examine the opposite breast.

◆ Begin in the area of the armpit and make straight rows of strips, using three pressures in each spot, not releasing the pressure as you spiral downward.

◆ Continue in the side-lying position until you reach your **nipple** and then **roll** to your **back;** remove your hand from your forehead and place on the bed**.**

◆ Continue to make rows of circles until you reach the middle of your breast bone. Examine the nipple with the same method. **Do not squeeze your nipple.**

◆ Assume side-lying position for the opposite breast exam and continue as above.

◆ Examine the lumpectomy breast or mastectomy area with the same thorough method of examination. Closely evaluate the scar area. Most recurrences are located in or near the incision area.

Lymph Node Examination

◆ Make a row of circles **under** your collar bone.

◆ Make a row of circles **above** your collar bone. To check in the depressed area, pull your shoulders upward, turn your face toward the side you are examining and place your fingers in the formed depression.

◆ Feel under each arm carefully for lymph node enlargement.

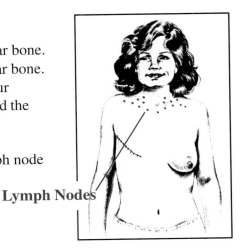

Lymph Nodes

Lymph nodes are pea-like areas in the lymphatic system that may become enlarged from the effects of the cancer. They will feel much like soft to hard June peas. Enlarged lymph nodes do not always indicate cancer but may occur from infection. A physician needs to be aware of any enlarged node finding so that the node(s) can be monitored. On your surgical side, the lymph nodes were partially or all removed from under the arm, but the ones under and above the collarbone still need to be monitored.

Visual Exam

Because some changes in the breast may not be felt but may be observed by closely looking at your breast, you need to perform a visual exam. Stand before a mirror in a bright light and observe your breast using these four different positions:

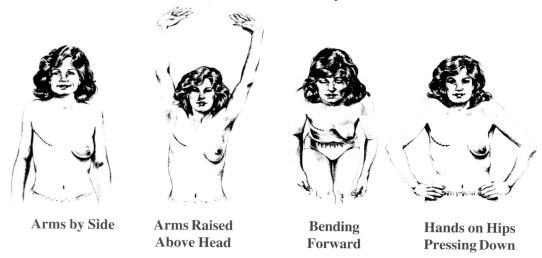

| **Arms by Side** | **Arms Raised Above Head** | **Bending Forward** | **Hands on Hips Pressing Down** |

In each position, observe your breast(s), looking straight on and then turn from side to side. If your breast(s) are large and sagging, you may need to lift the breast with your hand to observe the under area of the breast.

Visual exams allow you to check for any changes in the appearance of your breast(s). Some cancers do **not** form a hard lump, and the first change indicating cancer may be a visual change. Any visual changes observed should be reported to your physician for evaluation.

You will be looking for the following changes:

- ◆ Texture of your skin—may appear like an orange peeling (See Picture A)
- ◆ Color change (not including scar)—reddish or pinkish color or like a bruise on the skin

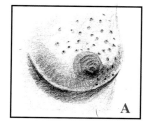

◆ Increase or decrease in the size of non-radiated breast

◆ Dimpling or pulling in of the skin (See Picture B)

◆ Inverted nipple (See Picture C)

◆ Crusty material or irritation around your nipple

◆ Bloody discharge from one nipple

◆ Bulging of skin

◆ Open sore or bump

◆ Difference in vein pattern on one breast—much larger veins or increased number of veins on one breast (See Picture D)

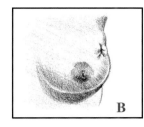

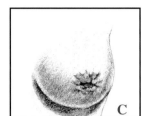

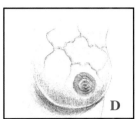

Remember

🖎 Breast self-exam is the best tool for monitoring for recurrence.

🖎 When you complete your monthly exam, congratulate yourself for taking an active part in guarding your health. Then forget about it until next month.

Mammograms After Surgery

The best defense against breast cancer is the breast self-exam. The second best defense is mammography. You probably had one performed to assist in diagnosing your breast cancer. You will continue to go on a regular basis for mammograms. If you had bilateral mastectomies, a prophylactic mastectomy or reconstruction, ask your physician for recommendations concerning regular mammograms. Some physicians may require more frequent mammograms of lumpectomy and mastectomy surgical patients the first several years. Other physicians feel yearly mammography is adequate surveillance. Your physician will tell you what schedule you will follow. Remember, even if you are under 35 your doctor may now want you to go for your mammograms on a yearly basis. Remind your doctor if your annual checkup does not include a mammogram. Remember to schedule your mammogram when your breast(s) is least tender. This is at the end of your period if you are pre-menopausal.

Make sure that your mammography facility has been certified by the U.S. Food and Drug Administration (FDA) as having met quality standards. If the facility does not have FDA certification, ask your physician to refer you to one that does.

Preparation for Mammogram

When you go for a mammogram, do not wear deodorant, perfume or powder on your upper body, as this could appear as a shadow or spot on your mammogram film. If you have had a painful mammogram in the past, stop caffeine intake several days prior or ask your physician about taking ibuprofen to reduce discomfort. If you change facilities for your mammogram, be sure to take your previous film for comparison.

Remember

❧ Have a **mammogram yearly**.

❧ Practice **breast self-exam monthly.**

❧ Have a doctor do a **clinical exam** at least yearly or more often, if necessary.

Using these three methods will help assure that a vigilant watch is being kept over your continued good health. **You need to practice all three methods of detection.**

Health Care After Cancer

During the first year after your treatment, you will be seen three or four times by your oncologist. If no problems arise, you will then progress to office visits several times a year. It is very important that you keep these visits with your doctor, even when you are feeling great.

Your physician will monitor your general health and order routine exams and screening tests to detect any recurrence or new problem. Regular blood work will be performed, and physical exams of the surgical area will take place on each visit. Bone scans, chest x-rays and other staging exams vary according to the schedule on which physicians repeat the exams. Continue to have a yearly pap smear and get your mammograms on a regular basis. You need to ask the following questions about your follow-up care:

◆ How often will I need to return for a checkup?

◆ Do I call and make the appointment, or does your office call me?

◆ What symptoms should I be aware of which might indicate a possible recurrence?

◆ What long lasting side effects of my treatment can I expect as normal?

◆ What should my arm and breast area look and feel like (painful, numb, tingling)?

◆ What changes might occur that I should consider dangerous and worthy of alerting you?

◆ Are there any special things that I should do or not do or that I should avoid (particular activities, medications, food)?

Dietary Changes for Better Health

If your physician does not recommend a special diet, you may wish to consider dietary changes that have proven beneficial in preventing many different health problems. Your hospital or clinic may have a nutritionist who can assist you in this process. Your goal should be to eat a balanced diet that promotes maintaining your ideal body weight while not making you feel hungry or deprived. Any diet which causes extreme hunger, or is psychologically depressing, is not healthy nor is it recommended for you. Avoid fad diets for weight reduction or maintenance.

Why Weight is Gained During Treatment

Weight gain experienced by some women during treatment for breast cancer has been linked to water retention from medications, taste changes from chemotherapy, relief from nausea achieved by keeping food in the stomach and an increase in eating patterns as a result of stress. Identifying the cause of any weight gain is helpful in addressing the problem.

Diet and Health

When we talk of diet, most people think of losing weight. Almost every woman at some time has gone on a diet to lose weight. However, what we eat not only affects our weight but, of even greater importance, it has a direct effect on our general health. Diet plays a major part in our health status and energy. As you are recovering from breast cancer, evaluate your eating habits and consider dietary changes as a healthy lifestyle choice for maximum health and energy.

Dietary fat has been linked to many diseases and is often the culprit for much unwanted weight and some illnesses. In the past, sugar has received the blame when fat was more of a common denominator. Therefore, a smart diet is monitoring what you eat to have a healthier life, and in the meantime you may lose unwanted pounds.

The Role of Dietary Fat

Findings regarding dietary fat include:

- Dietary fat has the ability to increase the level of the hormone estrogen which has been proven to stimulate some tumors.

- Dietary fat has been linked to higher cholesterol, which can lead to cardiovascular disease.

- Dietary fat has more calories than other type of nutrients (proteins and carbohydrates).

It is wise to lower anything that may promote disease and increase weight. For this reason, learn to count fat grams. Then learn to substitute healthful fats, mono and polyunsaturated fats such as safflower, sunflower and olive oils, in place of saturated fats such as animal, coconut and palm oils which cause an elevated cholesterol level.

Learn to:
- Read labels for percentages of fat content and fat grams per serving
- Read labels for the kinds of fat
- Select foods with healthy fats
- Limit the number of fat grams eaten daily

How to Find Your Daily Allowance of Fat

Authorities recommend that women eat no more than 25 percent of their daily calories from fat. To determine how many fat grams you can eat, divide the number of calories you consume a day by four (25 percent) or by five (20 percent).

Example:

2,000 calories a day divided by 4 = 500 calories a day from fat. Then divide the 500 calories from fat by 9 to get the grams of fat you can eat per day. 500 divided by 9 = 55 grams of fat per day.

Counting Fat Grams to Lose Weight

If you wish to lose weight, you may reduce your number of grams to a lower number but **do not go on a totally fat free diet. This is not healthy.** Between 15 and 25 percent of daily calories should come from dietary fat. Dietary fat contains essential daily nutrients.

Age	Weight	Fat Budget
25 - 50	110-130 lbs	65 grams
	130-150 lbs	75 grams
	150-170 lbs	85 grams
51 & up	110-130 lbs	55 grams
	130-150 lbs	65 grams
	150-170 lbs	75 grams

Now that you have determined the number of fat grams you can eat per day, find a fat gram chart and select the foods you may eat on a balanced diet that does not leave you feeling hungry or deprived.

Hints to Help You Maintain a Low Fat Diet
- Eat more chicken, turkey and fish instead of red meat (remove skin; do not fry).
- Broil or bake meat; cook with nonstick skillet and use cooking spray.
- Buy fat-free or low-fat salad dressings and mayonnaise.
- Buy low-fat cheese.

♦ Try frozen yogurt for dessert instead of ice cream.

♦ Look at fat grams in bread (most are low fat, but a croissant is high in fat).

♦ Eat more pasta and cereals.

♦ Eat more fresh fruit.

♦ Cook vegetables with little or no fat.

♦ Drink skim milk.

♦ Eat nonfat yogurt.

♦ Drink lots of water.

♦ Read all labels, watching for hidden fat.

Recommendations for Breast Cancer Patients

Dr. Henry Leis, a breast cancer surgeon, encourages his patients to adopt healthy eating habits for a lifetime. His advice to his breast cancer patients includes:

A low fat diet is recommended. Other factors of major importance include a high fiber, reduced calorie diet, avoidance of obesity, proper exercise, use of appropriate vitamins and minerals as supplements, limiting consumption of alcohol, salt-cured, smoked and nitrate-cured foods and reducing levels of environmental carcinogens.

"We are what we eat," and what we eat is one thing we can all control. A sensible approach of reducing dietary fat, adding additional fiber and eating a balanced diet can be a valuable tool in your recovery from breast cancer.

Remember

❧ Do not select a diet to lose weight; instead select a diet to create health.

❧ Diets which limit the amount of food eaten and create hunger are psychologically stressful and should always be avoided.

❧ Watching the amount of fat in your diet can improve your health and may cause a loss of weight.

❧ Do not allow three numbers on a bathroom scale to dictate how you feel about yourself.

❧ Concentrate on healthy eating habits, not numbers on a scale.

Staying Physically Fit

Recovery after breast cancer is also a time to consider an exercise program that suits you. Your hospital or clinic may offer or recommend exercise classes for breast cancer patients with a focus on regaining the range of motion of the surgical arm. These programs are very beneficial.

While these programs are helpful for your surgical recovery, you should also begin a program of regular exercise. The program you select does not need to be elaborate. You do not need to join a health club to begin. For example, walking is one of the most beneficial exercises. Consider your time and lifestyle to find an exercise that you will enjoy and participate in on a regular basis.

Benefits of Regular Exercise

Whatever exercise you select and consistently do will not only benefit you physically with higher energy levels, but will also serve to increase your psychological recovery from breast cancer. Exercise has been shown to improve both physical strength and psychological mood. Exercise also reduces pain by promoting the release of natural painkillers referred to as "endorphins" or "natural morphine" into the body. Regular exercise has been proven to help reduce depression.

Getting Started

If you are beginning an exercise program for the first time, check with your physician for approval and recommendations. You may want to ask a friend or a mate to join you in your new venture. Begin to slowly and gradually work up your endurance. Do not push yourself or exhaust your physical reserves; this is not healthy. Instead, look at this as a special time set aside to take care of your own needs and enjoy the activity. The rewards will be increased physical stamina and psychological well-being.

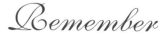

Remember

ﺑﺎ Exercise can elevate your mood and increase physical endurance.

ﺑﺎ Walking is one of the best forms of exercise.

ﺑﺎ Ask someone to join you; this will increase the likelihood that you will continue the program.

ﺑﺎ ﺑﺎ ﺑﺎ

Refer to the tear-out "Exercise Guidelines After Breast Cancer," located on page 183 - 184.

Chapter 11

Sexuality After Breast Cancer

*"Resuming sexual relations with my husband after surgery was not easy for me. I was not comfortable with my own sexuality and wasn't sure what I wanted or expected from my husband. Fortunately, he was more comfortable with this than I was. He very tenderly and lovingly helped me come to terms with this part of **our** recovery."*

~ Harriett Barrineau, survivor

Breast cancer has changed many things in your life. One of the potential changes may be in the area of your return to normal sexual functioning. Women share that their sexual attractiveness to their partner was of primary concern during their recovery. Many factors are involved in successfully adjusting to the change breast cancer has brought. It is helpful if you evaluate your present status and take steps to restore any areas that may not have returned to normal.

A woman's breasts play an important part in her femininity, and any breast surgery or disease will threaten her sense of being a female. This is a normal response. However, it is important that you take steps to incorporate these changes into a healthy perspective which allows you to return to your former state of functioning. Changes brought about by surgery are often related to your personal view of your new body self-image.

Your Body Image

One of the hardest and most important steps is viewing the incision area and the changed or missing breast. This is indeed difficult, but it is an essential step to recovery. Your mate most often will share your pain and loss and, when allowed to participate in this sensitive area, will have the doors opened to respond to your needs. Not allowing him to participate will build a wall of separation that will affect the sexual relationship.

Breasts add pleasure to the sexual relationship but are **not** essential for that pleasure to occur. It is not the loss of a breast that changes the relationship as much as the way you and your mate accept the loss. Facing the loss together and openly communicating about how your surgery may change your sexual relationship are the first steps in successfully adjusting. The earlier this is done, the smoother the transition to recovery.

Some women have shared that even though their mates had viewed the incision, they found difficulty in participating in sexual intimacy unclothed. This problem was solved by purchasing a lacy camisole which could be worn with or without a prosthesis. For some this served to preserve their feelings of femininity during the sexual relationship. Examine your feelings carefully as to what may be preventing you from resuming your sexual relationship with the one you love.

Side Effects of Treatment on Sexuality

During surgery or treatment, sexual functioning may be affected by fatigue or side effects from treatment. These are normal interruptions that will be time-limited and, when over, should not impair your former state of sexuality. Careful planning and management of your energy can allow you to plan for sexual intimacy during your treatments.

Side effects from chemotherapy or medications which cause menopausal symptoms may present problems which decrease sexual satisfaction. One change you may notice is in your sexual arousal. The reduction of the female hormones caused by medications during treatment naturally reduces sexual feelings. You may find sexual arousal diminished and that arousal takes longer. This does not mean that sexual feeling is gone, only that it requires more stimulation. Your mate needs to be aware of this fact. Often, a partner may assume that lack of response is rejection of them as a partner; they may not understand that it is a physical change that you are experiencing. Communicating honestly with your partner about this is the first step. You will need to allow more time to reach arousal sexually. Most mates are usually understanding when they have this problem shared with them.

Vaginal Dryness

One of the major side effects of treatment is vaginal dryness, which may result in painful intercourse and/or spotting after intercourse. Over-the-counter vaginal lubricants have proven helpful in reducing this problem (Replens® or Vagisil®). These products are applied **inside** the vagina on a **regular** schedule (not as a lubricant before intercourse) to restore and hold the internal moisture of the vagina. Try these products for several months. Some women have reported good results by massaging mineral oil into the **outside** vaginal tissues several times a week to reduce dryness.

Before intercourse, generously apply a water-soluble lubricant such as Astroglide® (highly recommended by patients) or K-Y Jelly®. Your physician needs to be informed of the problem if discomfort continues. Ask for additional recommendations to relieve the dryness.

Vaginal Infections

With an increase in vaginal dryness comes the potential for vaginal infections. The most common one is caused by a fungus that women commonly refer to as a "yeast" infection. This infection is identified by having a thick, white discharge which resembles cottage cheese and causes extreme itching and swelling in the vaginal area. Over-the-counter medications are available and usually are very helpful in managing the condition. If the problem is recurrent, it may be helpful if you have your partner treated with the cream while you are being treated with the cream or suppositories. If the condition continues after this treatment, a physician should be notified. Other types of vaginal infections may be the reason, and the cause needs to be identified and treated.

Talk to Your Physician

Openly communicate with your physician about **any** physical problem you are experiencing. Some women feel that the physicians they are seeing after breast cancer are only interested in saving their lives and not in their daily life functions. This is **NOT** true. Physicians are well aware that quality of life is one of the main components for a successful recovery. Because they do not ask about the sexuality problems does not mean that they will not discuss and help you with any of your concerns.

Surgery has not changed you. You may experience some new problems after your surgery and treatment for cancer which challenge you and your mate. But you are still the same loving person your mate selected, and surgery does not change that fact. Many couples share that surgery brought them closer together, and the sexual relationship was enhanced because of the realization of how valuable they were to each other.

Restoring Sexual Function

- ◆ Have I allowed my mate to see my scar? Am I still hiding in the closet to change clothes?
- ◆ Have I talked openly about my fear that our relationship will change?
- ◆ Have I expressed my desire for our sexual functioning not to be affected?
- ◆ Have I shared openly about what is physically comfortable or uncomfortable during intimacy since my surgery?
- ◆ Am I honest when I am physically fatigued and would like to be held and cuddled without intercourse?
- ◆ Have I explained that, when I do not feel up to the sexual act, I am not rejecting my mate, but I need time to adjust or it is a side effect (fatigue) of my treatment?
- ◆ Have I planned a special time and saved energy for the sexual relationship to be resumed?

◆ Have I been honest and asked for family assistance with household duties during treatments to allow me more time and energy for pleasurable events?

◆ When I have problems, such as a dry vagina or painful intercourse due to treatment side effects, do I talk with my physician about how to manage the problems?

◆ Have I had my body image restored with a well-fitted prosthesis or had/or planned for reconstruction?

◆ If interested in reconstructive surgery, have I talked to a physician and received the information needed to make a decision?

◆ If I am having problems adjusting to my body image or sexuality, have I asked to speak to a counselor?

◆ Have I asked my treatment team or called the American Cancer Society for information on sexuality after cancer?

◆ Have I treated myself to a feminine treat to enhance my feeling of femininity after surgery (such as perfume, an item of clothing, or a new haircut)?

Readjustment in the area of sexual functioning is a most common occurrence in breast cancer patients. There are many things you can do. There is help you can receive to assist the return to your normal sexual role. Don't allow changes to occur without reaching out to your physician, nurse or support group to ask for information and, if needed, counseling. The earlier you address these problems, the easier they are to solve. Educational material is available, and trained counselors can help you with the transition.

Birth Control After Breast Cancer

It is necessary to discuss with your physician what type of birth control to use after your surgery. Chemotherapy usually stops your menstrual periods, and they may or may not return after the treatments are completed. If you are near menopause, they may never come back. However, if you are young, they may return. For some women, several years may go by before normal menstruation begins again. Because you may be fertile (able to conceive a child) **before evidence of a menstrual period**, you may want to discuss with your physician the type of birth control which is suitable for you. Do **not** take any **oral contraceptives** (birth control pills) without talking to your oncologist. Alternate methods of birth control will be recommended according to the type of treatment you receive.

One Note on Tamoxifen

The anti-estrogen drug, Tamoxifen (Nolvadex®), may **increase** ovulation (release of the egg from the ovary) when therapy is started. After receiving Tamoxifen, women may be more

98

fertile, and multiple births have been reported. **Contraception is recommended.** Discuss with your physician what types of contraception are most suitable and the length of time recommended for use to prevent pregnancy.

Pregnancy After Breast Cancer

Most young women want to know if they can have a child after their breast cancer treatment is completed. Women have had healthy babies after their treatment. A woman's eggs are all present, in her ovaries, at the time of her birth. Chemotherapy does **not** damage the eggs, because eggs are not dividing cells.

However, there are **many variables** to be considered in making the decision. You need to discuss the desire with your health care team. The health-related decision from a physician's point of view may include an evaluation of the following:

- Cell type of cancer
- How difficult the original cancer was to diagnose (for example, if it did not show up on a mammogram or you had no lump, then surveillance for a recurrence may be more difficult during pregnancy)
- Ductal involvement (in situ or invasive)
- Size of tumor
- Lymph node involvement
- Nuclear grade, aggressiveness of tumor
- Evidence of spread of cancer to other parts of your body
- Hormone dependence (estrogen, progesterone)
- Type of treatment required to initially treat your cancer (chemotherapy, stem cell, bone marrow)
- Response to initial treatment
- Time elapsed since treatment

If you are in your child-bearing years and would like to have a baby, discuss this with your **team** of physicians. Only when **all** the details of your particular cancer type, spread and previous treatment are understood can appropriate advice be given.

Pregnancy does not cause breast cancer. However, if pregnant, some treatments may have to be precluded if you have a recurrence. The final decision is **individual** and rests on the degree of **risk** you are willing to take to bring a child into the world. It is important to explore and gather the facts to make an informed decision. Your team of physicians will gladly provide you with the medical facts of your diagnosis and treatment to help you with the decision.

Remember

ভ‍ু The key to preventing changes in the sexual relationship is open, honest communication with your mate.

ভ‍ু Viewing the incision site as early as possible removes the greatest obstacle to restoring the relationship.

ভ‍ু Seek help from your health care team for any physical problems you experience. Ask about the need for contraception. Discuss with your physician any future desire to have a child.

ভ‍ু You are still the same loving person your mate selected. Breast cancer does not change that fact.

Chapter 12

Monitoring Your Mental Recovery

"My physical recovery went well. At first, it seemed, so was my mental and emotional state. After three or four months, things began to change. I knew people still cared, but the initial interest and concern began to wane. I was still surrounded by so much love, yet, I was feeling totally alone."

~ Harriett Barrineau, survivor

The unexpected diagnosis of breast cancer can serve as a threat to a woman's life, self-esteem, body image, sexuality, social life and career. Many confusing emotions accompany the diagnosis as these threats are individually worked into her life; however, most women manage to cope successfully. Tears are natural and an expected response, just as occasional periods of depression are natural. This natural depression after a loss is called a **reactive depression.** Scattered throughout the months after your surgery and during treatment, you will have periods of feeling down. Therefore, reactive depression is a common emotional state after a loss and is expected after the diagnosis of breast cancer. However, it is essential to understand the difference between a normal reaction of feeling depressed and clinical depression, which requires intervention by health professionals.

Reactive Depression

In the future, sometimes for no known reason or because a situation has upset you, you may find yourself feeling depressed. If the feeling lasts for several days and you begin to feel better, this is a normal reaction (reactive depression) after a major loss in your life.

It is helpful to realize that these periodic feelings of sadness, which last for several days, may occur in the future. However, these periods of depression should be short-term. These often occur on anniversary dates of diagnosis, surgery or treatments and are referred to as **"anniversary reactions."** These dates may bring back vividly all the memories and feelings

101

experienced during these events in the past. This same depression may occur around the time for a return visit to your physician for a **check-up** after breast cancer. We refer to this normal reactive depression as **"check-up anxiety."** Most breast cancer patients experience some degree of anxiety during the **anniversary** of their diagnosis or surgery. **Anniversary reactions** are **normal**, as is check-up anxiety, but anticipating and planning can significantly reduce the emotional strain. Another time many women feel depressed is at the conclusion of all their chemotherapy or radiation treatments. This depression is referred to as **post-treatment depression** and is very common.

It can be helpful if you anticipate these times and plan your activities to accommodate for your "blue" feelings. Plan a special time away from your routine duties to do something special, spend time with friends or arrange a light schedule of work.

However, some women may have problems incorporating this major loss into their lives. Their depression and tears do not cease but continue long after surgery and treatments are completed. These periods may occur often or remain as a constant companion. This may signal a need for additional help in making the adjustment psychologically.

Depression Which Needs Intervention

It is helpful if you recognize the difference between a normal reactive depression to your diagnosis and one that signals clinical depression (depression that needs professional intervention). This is a serious condition with real symptoms that affect both the mind and the body. Symptoms are prolonged and severe and increasingly incapacitate your ability to return to normal functioning. The positive fact is that clinical depression usually responds positively to counseling and medication. Ninety percent of people who seek help find their treatment successful. This type of depression is more than just feeling "down" or "blue" after a loss or disappointment

The first step in distinguishing the difference between feeling blue and clinical depression is to know the warning signs and not feel uncomfortable about seeking appropriate help. Women can be helped to overcome depression and live a normal, healthy life. "Feeling blue" or periodic depression means that one may feel sad but can still enjoy and look forward to parts of life, such as a family gathering, a movie or seeing a friend. **Clinical depression**, on the other hand, is often manifested by:

◆ Continuous (week after week) feelings of sadness during or after surgery and treatment

◆ Social withdrawal from friends or family

◆ Feelings of worthlessness

◆ Excessive feelings of guilt

◆ Excessive feelings of fear of the future

◆ Being very slow in physical movement or speech

102

◆ Constant jitters or nervousness with no apparent reason

◆ Low energy level; feeling tired all the time

◆ Inability to make decisions

◆ Negative thinking, constantly angry or mistrustful

◆ Imaginary health problems

◆ Obsessions about health and cancer

◆ General disinterest in food or eating excessively

◆ Disinterest in work or day-to-day activities (things which used to interest you)

◆ Disinterest in intimacy or sex

◆ Insomnia (inability to sleep, waking early or being unable to go to sleep)

◆ Hypersomnia (sleeping too much, wanting to sleep all the time)

◆ Suicidal thoughts

If you find that you are experiencing several of these symptoms (some experts say five) for a period of two weeks or longer during or after treatment completion, **your physician should be notified.** If you have suicidal thoughts and feel that death would be an easy choice, **please call your physician or nurse immediately.**

Treatment for Depression

Depression may be treated in several ways. For mild cases, counseling may be all that is needed. Counseling identifies weaknesses in coping skills and works to strengthen them. Often, talking to an understanding person accomplishes much for a depressed person. Medication may be needed to assist the process. Antidepressants, medications used to treat depression, are often prescribed and generally take up to two weeks to provide positive results. A nutritious diet and regular exercise have also been proven to be beneficial in reducing depression and stress. A professional can evaluate an individual and determine the most appropriate type of help.

If you are experiencing depression, know that this is **not** a sign of weakness. Many breast cancer patients have a struggle adjusting. This is a legitimate condition that is experienced by many people after a major crisis or loss. Breast cancer patients also have to deal with hormonal fluctuations. These hormonal fluctuations, brought about by cancer treatment, may cause radical changes in emotions.

After breast cancer, most depression persists for a **short** period of time, and short-term counseling or medication can help you through this period of adjustment. **Identifying and seeking help is the first step** to resolving the problem of depression. Most patients respond well to counseling or medication. **If you are experiencing depression, consult your physician.** Asking for appropriate help is a **sign of strength,** not weakness.

Remember

- Depression is not a sign of weakness.

- Depression is common after a major loss or crisis.

- Most depression is generally short-term and responds to counseling and medication.

- Seeking help for depression is a sign of strength.

It's Okay To Cry

Crying is a very acceptable and healthy expression of grief.
Crying shows how deeply you feel and how much you care.
Crying helps relieve the tension that has built up inside of you.
Crying is an expression of deep contrition and of unspeakable love.
Crying speaks for you when you cannot find the words.
Crying helps you to recover your physical and emotional strength.
Crying is not the mark of weakness, but of power.
Crying allows grief to be done in a constructive way.
Crying enables you to cope with a significant loss.
Crying is a way of communicating with your humanity.
Crying ventilates feelings of anger and hurt.
~ Encouragement Ministries

"Tears are salve on our wounds." ~ Nicholas Wolterstorff

❧ ❧ ❧

Refer to the tear-outs, "My Prayer During Breast Cancer," "What Cancer Can't Do" and "Remember," at the back of the book.

Chapter 13

Health Insurance and Employment Issues

"Nothing prepared me for the magnitude of the responsibility I would have in seeing to it that I received the insurance benefits to which I was entitled. I was overwhelmed by the number of bills I received following surgery. Good record keeping was essential."

~ Harriett Barrineau, survivor

When you are diagnosed with breast cancer, if you have health insurance, inform your provider and ask for guidelines for filing or payment of claims. The following questions may need to be clarified. Some of the answers may be found in your insurance policy manuals.

- Is there a need for second opinions for procedures?

- Do I need pre-approval for hospital admissions?

- How do I file claims?

- What is the name of a person at the company who can answer questions about my case?

- What is the amount of the deductible, if any, required before claims are paid?

- Are there any limits imposed on the amount paid for surgery, chemotherapy, radiation therapy or reconstruction?

- What is the policy regarding coverage for new treatments or treatments considered "experimental" (autologous stem cell therapy, autologous bone marrow treatments, etc.)? Are there limits on what amounts will be paid?

- What is the policy regarding coverage for a permanent prosthesis? If delayed reconstruction is considered, will it pay for both, or does one exclude payment for the other?

Record Keeping for Reimbursement

After breast cancer, it is very important that you take steps to receive payment for services covered under your insurance. Many women find this task overwhelming emotionally or physically. Often, a mate or a friend will volunteer to perform this job for you. Ask for assistance in this area. Records you keep will make the task much easier.

Taking the Hassle Out of Record Keeping

- Keep calendar records of all appointments (a pocket calendar for this purpose is helpful).

- Write on the calendar the physician visited, procedures performed and medications purchased.

- Provide physicians with appropriate information and forms for filing claims.

- Ask for copies of **all** charges at the time of service or ask to have copies mailed to you.

- **Keep** copies of all charges from appointments or services **in one place** (a box, a notebook or file folder).

- Periodically check to see if payment is appropriately made to medical providers.

- If problems arise, request your health care facility or provider to help you understand or assist you in providing information for adequate repayment.

- Call your insurance providers and talk with a claims representative. Offer additional records or assistance for getting information from your medical providers.

- Keep all premiums current; **do not allow your insurance to lapse.**

Insurance After Diagnosis

After any major illness, insurance is more difficult to obtain. For this reason, keep all premium payments current. If you decide to change jobs, be sure that you will be covered under the new employer's insurance program **before** making a decision. If you have private insurance or coverage through your employment, be very alert to these areas before making major decisions.

Financial Assistance

If your illness is going to be a financial burden to you, ask to speak to the social worker in the cancer treatment center. Social workers are trained to help you with the social issues of your illness, including helping you secure financial help for needed medical services. There are various services available, but you will need to apply for them. The earlier you can make this need known, the more effective the social work team can be in helping you file the forms.

People often feel embarrassed to ask for help and postpone the issue. Many people find an unexpected illness drains their financial reserves. **You are not alone. Ask for help early.**

Employment Issues During Treatment

Breast cancer surgery and treatment will require some time away from your job. Most employers are very understanding and offer their support during this time. You will need to give notice of your absence and expected time away from your job.

Occasionally, however, a breast cancer patient will be discriminated against because of illness. If you have reasons to believe that your employer has treated you unfairly because of your illness, there are laws which protect you. There are federal laws and varying state laws which offer protection against discrimination or unfair practices. Listed in the reference section of this book are names and telephone numbers which you can call to receive information on how to best manage your situation.

What Do You Tell Your Friends?

It is necessary for you to decide how much to tell your employer, fellow employees and friends about the details of your illness. Some women are very open about their illness and treatments. Others feel that this is a private matter and would rather not share the details with everyone. Decide what you wish for others to know. It is helpful if you inform your support partner or family members so that your wishes can be carried out when people call or drop by.

You do not have to constantly share your "illness story" with others if this makes you uncomfortable. A simple reply of "I appreciate your concern, but right now I am not up to talking about it. Thank you for understanding," allows you the right not to tell. You need to communicate, but you do not need to feel that you have to talk with everyone. It may be helpful to allow family members to answer the phone and screen your calls if you would rather not talk. Plan to do what best suits your particular personality.

Remember

❧ Simple record keeping will help take the hassle out of insurance filing.

❧ Recruit someone to help with record keeping.

❧ Keep your insurance premiums current.

❧ Do not change jobs unless you know you will be covered by the new insurance.

❧ If you experience discrimination on the job, seek assistance from professionals.

❧ ❧ ❧

As Survivors,
we accept responsibility for our
own lives. We refuse to blame
others, God or fate for our
misfortune. We do not allow our
misfortune to be an excuse for
personal unhappiness. Instead we
take action to transform the
unfortunate into a catalyst for good.
We change whatever impairs us
into a tool for personal growth.

Chapter 14

Facing the Future After Breast Cancer

*"I consider myself a survivor, not a victim.
I think about recurrence, but it no longer consumes me.
I do not fear death, nor do I fear life after having had breast cancer.
My life will never be the same as before,
but any negatives breast cancer has brought
have been matched by positives."*

~ Harriett Barrineau, survivor

No woman would ever choose to have breast cancer. Breast cancer changes your life, and there are things that will never be the same after diagnosis. Yet, many have shared that the breast cancer experience added a new dimension to their lives—one that allowed them to enjoy life even more than before.

Recovery from breast cancer is a gradual process mentally, just as it is physically. The physical healing usually comes long before the psychological healing. Steps to psychological recovery must be taken by you on your own timetable. Some women are eager to put the experience behind them, while others need time to absorb the impact of the changes that cancer brings. Only you can decide what is best for you. Just as your treatment team has plans for you to recover physically, **you need to chart a mental recovery plan**.

High Risk Relatives

Your diagnosis of breast cancer has changed many things in your family, particularly the fact that your daughters, sisters and mother are now considered at **"high risk"** for the disease. This is a term that terrorizes thousands of women each year after a family diagnosis of breast cancer. However, being considered high risk may be a **blessing.** Because of a family diagnosis of breast cancer, women and their physicians will watch their breasts and health more carefully. If cancer should occur, close monitoring should find it in an early stage when it is most treatable. Women with no history may lack the motivation to be diligent and ignore guidelines for early detection and screening, resulting in late detection.

What Does "High Risk" Really Mean?

High risk is **not** an absolute fact. A history of breast cancer does **not** mean your first degree relatives will have the disease. It is more like a yellow light, a warning to be cautious. A family history is **no** reason for panic, but it should be a motivation to learn steps for protection and early detection. Based on current information, approximately **10 percent** or fewer breast cancers have a family connection. Family members' risks increase about **two** to **three** percent if your cancer was past your menopause. If your cancer was before menopause, or if you had cancer in both breasts, the risk is **four** to **five** times greater.

It will be helpful to your family members if you address their fears with accurate information regarding their risks. Most people overestimate and often become paralyzed with unfounded fear. Information can be obtained from your physician, the American Cancer Society, the National Cancer Institute and other sources listed in the reference section of this book.

The Following Positive Steps Can be Taken to Protect Your Relatives:

- They can find a physician who is aware of the family history of breast cancer and will monitor their breast health closely with thorough clinical exams of their breasts.

- You can give them the name of the type of breast cancer you had so that this information can be passed along to their physicians. Some cancers with a familial characteristic may show up in the relative with very similar characteristics to your cancer. (Example: if your cancer was found on mammography, or if your cancer did not show up on mammography, this will be helpful information for their surveillance.)

- They can learn how to perform the breast self-exam from a health professional and practice it monthly.

- They need to follow guidelines for mammography screening. Some physicians recommend that daughters begin their screening ten years younger than the age at which a mother's breast cancer was detected.

- They can learn controllable life-style factors that have been implicated in contributing to breast cancer and other diseases, such as diet (especially high fat) and various carcinogens. They can take the necessary steps to modify their diets and life-styles.

110

◆ They can seek support from health professionals in understanding "high risk status," take steps against misinformation and learn the latest information on fighting the disease.

Remember

❧ "High risk" may be a blessing because of awareness and closer surveillance for your family members.

❧ Being "high risk" does not mean a woman will definitely have breast cancer.

❧ Family members can take positive steps to monitor their own breast health and master the fear of being "high risk."

Survivorship Attitudes

In my work with breast cancer survivors, I have listened to hundreds of breast cancer stories. As a care giver who intervened throughout the entire breast cancer experience, I shared their tears, fears and triumphs. From all of this I have observed and refined what I feel are attitudes of survivorship—attitudes which can help build an even richer life after a breast cancer diagnosis. These attitudes are not new. There are no secrets revealed here. Yet, somehow in the midst of a crisis it can be helpful if someone reminds you of what has worked in the past for others. Survivorship attitudes lead others to happiness "in spite of" the event which has paid an unexpected visit to their lives. As you read through this list, think of how these attitudes may help to add a sense of control and joy back to your life.

Suggestions From Other Women That Have Proven Beneficial
◆ Demystify cancer. Learn the facts about cancer. Correct your misconceptions.
◆ Do not concentrate on the "what ifs." The past is the past, and yesterday cannot be changed. Concentrate, rather, on what **you can do now.**
◆ Participate in your treatment decisions. Get answers to your questions before you agree to surgery or treatments. This is your life and your breast(s), and you will feel much more in control when you express your needs regarding treatment decisions.
◆ Do not suppress your emotions. Cry when you need to, and talk about your experience. Grieve your loss. Talk to someone you can trust about your feelings and fears. It may be necessary to find this person outside of the family unit.

- Identify your fears. Write them down and take action to disarm them.

- Plan to turn loose all anger, bitterness and hatred toward people and events in the past. Anger and hate are "joy robbers." Let it go. Refuse to let it use any of your energy or occupy your thoughts. Don't live in the yesterdays of your life. Live today. Replace bad attitudes with those that lay a foundation for health . . .love, peace and joy.

- Know that you may not be able to choose what happens to your body but that you can choose what happens in your **mind.** Be the master of your thoughts and refuse to camp in the land of despair and hopelessness. Negative thoughts are normal but you can choose to acknowledge them and take steps to think on more positive aspects of your life. Decide what happens in your mind: choose hope; think positively; think gratefully about what others have done for you; think lovingly.

- Learn focused thinking. Concentrate on the things that you have control over and can change. **Do not focus** on things that you have **no power over or cannot change.**

- Participate in a support group. Find a group which provides education as well as support. Women who attend support groups tend to adjust better than those who do not reach out.

- Use your spiritual faith as a source of strength and a place to find answers and give meaning to the hard questions of life.

- Allow your family and friends to participate in your recovery by helping you as needed. Tell them what you need. Don't make them guess. It is therapeutic for them to feel needed.

- Offer outside support resources to your family, such as written materials and support groups, to help them understand and adjust to your diagnosis. Encourage them to reach out.

- Form a partnership with your treatment team in battling the disease. Learn how you can best participate for maximum response during treatment.

- Communicate openly and honestly with your treatment team. They need your input.

- Remember, you are the only one that knows what is really happening to your body and what **tools you need to recover**.

- Stop long enough to say "thank you" or "I appreciate you" to those who are your care givers. Like you, they need to know they are appreciated and valued. Being a care giver is not always easy, and most people forget to share what they feel.

◆ Eat healthy. Exercise regularly. Physically rest when necessary. Get adequate sleep.

◆ Take time to do the things that make you feel good, whatever they may be. Plan you own fun times. Don't wait for happiness to come. Go and find it!

◆ Surround yourself with the things you love . . . music, books, pets, whatever makes you smile.

◆ Don't revert to covering your anxiety with alcohol or drugs. This only postpones your psychological recovery and can lead to depression.

◆ Plan. Decide when and what you are going to do to make this a time of intensive growth as a person. Chart new courses for yourself that you have always wanted to pursue. Take a class, read a long book, take a trip, plant a flower garden or whatever you have always wanted to do "when I have time." This will give you new energy and facilitate recovery.

◆ Acknowledge that there are going to be days when things don't go well, and you don't feel well physically or psychologically. But remember to reach out, ask for help if needed, and know that "this, too, will pass." Don't try to be a "superwoman" emotionally.

◆ Prepare yourself for those emotionally trying days (of treatment, medical tests or anniversary dates) with a physically and emotionally stress-free schedule as much as possible. Recruit a friend to share this time or plan a special treat for yourself to soften the experience.

◆ Follow your physician's guide for medical monitoring after cancer. Keep your appointments, perform the breast self-exam monthly, get your mammograms, but **don't** make a "career" out of cancer. Don't let it dominate your thoughts and actions.

◆ Give back to others out of your experience. Many women can benefit from your learning experience during breast cancer treatment. Find the best expression for your talents. Consider becoming a **Reach To Recovery** volunteer and visit other patients or join in fund raisers or activities to support other patients. Find your way to pass on the support you received.

◆ Look at the breast cancer experience as the "caution light" in your life that allowed you to slow down and examine your real needs and wishes for the future.

Remember

❧ You are **not** a **statistic.** You are an **individual**. Do not look at your future purely from statistical tables. If only one person has ever beaten the odds, you have the right to become the second.

❧ Survivorship is mostly attitude . . . the attitude that "I CAN." Become the best survivor ever! Start today to build the tomorrow that you desire.

Breast cancer is an unwelcome visitor in any woman's life. You have found yourself forced to embrace an unwanted enemy. Yet, even in the midst of this frightening and often lonely experience, you do have the capacity to find new strength and work through the challenge. Like thousands of other women, you can become a triumphant survivor. My love and best wishes for a happy and healthy future.

Judy Kneece

"All of us have heard the saying, 'Take time to stop and smell the roses.'
This became very important to me after my cancer diagnosis.
Someone told me to look upon all this as my 'wake-up call to live.'
That was excellent advice. I appreciate life more now. I take time for myself now.
I am bolder about talking to others about good breast health care.
I'm trying new things in life. Having breast cancer
and coming face to face with my own mortality
is the hardest thing I've ever had to deal with.
No, breast cancer is not an unconquerable enemy.
However, your entire life will be changed by cancer.
*You won't believe it now, but good **will** come out of this experience—if you let it."*

~ Harriett Barrineau, survivor

❧ ❧ ❧

Refer to the tear-out worksheet, "Personal Plan for Recovery,"
located at the back of the book.

114

Appendix A

Understanding Diagnostic Tests

Blood Counts

Your doctor will monitor your blood counts by drawing blood from your finger, arm or implanted vascular port on a regular basis. This evaluates how you respond to the effects of chemotherapy, monitors for infections and detects changes in your blood chemistry. The main counts monitored will be:

- **Red blood cells (RBCs)** which carry oxygen to all parts of your body
- **White blood cells (WBCs)** which combat infection and provide immunity
- **Platelets** which determine how your blood will clot
- **Electrolytes** (potassium, magnesium, sodium, chloride, glucose and carbon dioxide)
- **Hemoglobin (iron)** the portion of the red blood cells (RBCs) that attaches to oxygen

Remind the technician drawing the sample **not** to use your surgical arm. If you had bilateral mastectomies, the technician will need to use sterile procedures to reduce the potential for infection.

Normal Values	
Red blood cells (RBCs)	4.2-5.4 million/mm³
White blood cells (WBCs)	5,000-10,000/mm³
Hemoglobin (Hgb)	12-16 g/dl
Platelets	150,000-400,000/mm³

Bone Scan

Your physician may order a bone scan to evaluate and determine which stage of breast cancer was found. This scan is one of the most commonly performed nuclear medicine procedures used to determine if cancer has spread to the bones. The test is routinely ordered by physicians to stage your cancer.

On the day of the scan, you will have a radioactive substance intravenously injected into your arm, similar to having your blood drawn. This will cause little discomfort, and no side effects should occur from the injected material. In order for the radioactive substance to get to the bone, you will have a wait of several hours (one to three) before the actual testing will begin. You will need to drink several glasses of water after your injection to help eliminate, through your kidneys, any of the substance not picked up by the bones. You may want to take something to read, or you may leave and come back to the clinic for the scan. There is no other preparation on your part.

The scan requires you to lie on a table as a machine moves above your body from head to toe. You will be asked to empty your bladder before the test. You will be dressed, and there is no discomfort unless you find it difficult to lie flat and still. The scan may require as long as one hour to complete. The machine will scan your body and produce images of the structure of your bones. This machine does not give off radiation to your body. The only radiation you receive is in the injected substance, which is equal to the amount of radiation received from a regular diagnostic x-ray. An increased amount of the radioactive substance in an area of the bones, referred to as a "hot spot," may indicate an abnormality that the physician will further evaluate.

The radioactive substance given is of insufficient radioactivity to necessitate taking any special radiation precautions. The radioactive material will be excreted through the urine within 24 hours. You are not a risk to your family members during this time. The information gathered by the scan will be translated into x-ray pictures and a report sent to your physician.

Computed Tomography (CT) Scan

The CT scan, an advanced x-ray technique, enables your physician and the radiologist to view the bones and organs of your head and body in fine detail. This diagnostic procedure allows an earlier and faster diagnosis than the traditional x-ray. The test is performed inside a large x-ray tube. Pictures are taken in rapid sequence and sent to a computer to be studied by the physician and the radiologist.

The part of your body to be examined determines how you will need to prepare for the scan. In some cases, you may be asked not to eat or drink anything prior to the test. You may be given a contrast agent (radioactive substance) to drink or it may be injected into your vein to help highlight certain body parts. Tell the technologist if you have been given a contrast agent before, if you are allergic to seafood, iodine or other medications, if you have kidney problems, if you are diabetic or if you are pregnant.

You will be asked to lie very still on a table for the duration of the scan. A built-in communications system enables two-way conversation between you and the technologist at anytime during the scan. The automated table will move you into the scanner's x-ray tube, a donut-shaped ring, to take pictures of your body. You can expect to hear mechanical noises from the scanner as it takes pictures and collects data.

Inform your physician if you are claustrophobic (afraid of enclosed places). A medication may be given prior to the test to relax you during the scan. If you receive medication, you will need to bring a family member or a friend to drive you home. If you have difficulty lying down and being still because of pain, you may wish to take pain medication prior to the scan.

If you are given a contrast agent, it will naturally leave your body within 24 hours. You should increase the amount of water you drink to help get rid of the agent from your body through your kidneys. CT scans give off no more radiation than a series of regular x-ray studies, and you are not radioactive. This is a painless procedure.

Liver Scan

A liver scan allows your physician to check for structural changes in your liver. Prior to the test, you will be injected with a radioactive contrast agent through a vein. The contrast agent travels to the liver and allows special pictures to be taken, showing the uptake of the contrast agent. Approximately 30 minutes after the agent is administered, you will lie down on a table while a special instrument, a gamma ray detector (Geiger counter), is passed over your abdomen. You will be asked to change positions so all surfaces of the liver can be seen. The gamma ray detector will record the uptake of the contrast agent in the liver, and pictures will be made of the liver. These pictures will then be studied by your physicians.

The contrast agent will naturally leave your body in hours. You are not exposed to large amounts of radioactive material in this test. After the test is completed, you may resume your normal activities. This scanning procedure is completely painless.

Magnetic Resonance Imaging (MRI)

An MRI may be ordered by your doctor to detect the spread of cancer to other parts of your body. A strong magnet using radio frequency waves produces pictures to be read by a radiologist.

There are no restrictions on eating, drinking or taking your medications prior to the test. If you have a pacemaker, inform the physician in charge. You **cannot** have an MRI done because the magnetic field would damage the pacemaker. If you have internal metal clips or artificial heart valves, you **cannot** have an MRI performed. You will also need to inform the staff if you are claustrophobic (afraid or nervous in small spaces) so they can medicate you to relax you during the test. If you are claustrophobic, you will need to bring a friend or family member to drive you home because of sedation from the medication.

You will be placed on a table that enters a machine which looks like a long tube with open ends. You will need to lie very still during the test. The procedure is painless and requires from 15 minutes to one hour, according to the area(s) being examined. The reports will be sent to your doctor within several days.

117

Methylene Blue Dye Localization

This procedure may be required when a suspicious area on a mammogram cannot be felt by the surgeon. The dye is inserted into the suspicious area of the breast to color the area in order to aid the surgeon with the procedure. Using x-ray as a guide, the radiologist inserts the dye by injection with a needle. The surgeon removes the tissue stained by the dye. The tissue is sent to pathology for analysis. Needle localization biopsy or methylene blue are two procedures used to help the surgeon locate suspicious areas during surgery.

Needle Localization Biopsy

Needle localization biopsy is needed when a suspicious place shows up on a mammogram and cannot be felt with the hands. You will be taken to x-ray where the radiologist will place your breast under a mammography machine. While the breast is visualized, the radiologist will insert a wire into the spot that was seen previously on your mammogram. The insertion of the wire can be uncomfortable. However, analgesic medications can be given to alleviate the discomfort. The wire will be taped to your chest after a series of pictures confirm accurate placement. You will then be taken to surgery for the removal of the suspicious area. The removed tissue will be sent to the pathologist for diagnosis.

Stereotactic Needle Biopsy

If a suspicious area that cannot be felt or is very small is seen on a mammogram, stereotactic breast biopsy (Mammotest) may be used to biopsy the area. This biopsy procedure is performed using a mammography table, a biopsy needle and the guidance of a computer. This test, a new alternative to surgical biopsy, is done without the discomfort, risk of disfigurement and expense of surgery. The procedure takes approximately 45 minutes to perform, and most patients return to their normal activities within a few hours.

Your breast will be compressed with a special mammography machine while stereo x-ray pictures are taken at angles. After the suspicious area has been identified, the radiologist enters information into a computer that calculates where the needle should be injected. The area of the breast to be biopsied is deadened with a local anesthetic. An instrument moves the biopsy needle in position and at a rapid rate of speed removes a sample of the suspicious tissue. If the suspicious area is a cyst and needs aspiration, the needle will be placed into the area and confirmed with x-rays before the aspiration begins. Because stereotactic biopsy uses a needle, damage to nearby tissue is minimal, unlike surgery which may cause scarring to the breast. When the biopsy is complete, a Band-Aid® will be placed over the biopsy site, and you may return to your normal activities. You may shower the same day of the biopsy.

The biopsy sample will be sent to the pathology lab for evaluation. The pathologist will send the referring physician a report stating if the biopsy was malignant or benign. Consult your physician regarding how and when you can expect to receive the biopsy results.

Infection is rare with stereotactic biopsy. However, there is a small possibility a hematoma (a collection of blood under the skin) may develop. If this occurs, inform your physician so this information can be recorded in your medical records. This area may later show up on mammography as a change in your breast tissues.

Ultrasound

Ultrasonography, commonly referred to as an ultrasound, is a harmless test utilizing high-frequency sound waves that are sent out from a transducer, a microphone-like instrument. As the transducer moves over the breast tissue, the sound waves are bounced back to a sensor within the instrument where a picture on a monitor shows the internal structures of the breasts. These pictures, unlike a mammogram, use no radiation and allow the physician to observe the breast structures in motion. This test does not require any surgery or needles There is no advance preparation on your part, and the test is painless.

Ultrasounds are usually used when an abnormality has been found in a breast on a mammography exam. The test determines if the suspicious area is solid tissue or is a cyst, filled with fluid. The ultrasound accurately locates and correctly distinguishes the makeup of a lump more than 95 percent of the time. Breast cysts are easily identified by ultrasound, which often prevents unnecessary surgery for abnormal breast lumps that cannot be felt. It is also a very useful diagnostic tool for lumps found in pregnant women, for whom mammography is not advised.

The guidance of ultrasound visualization of the lump can aid the physician in accurate location of the area for withdrawal of the fluid from a cyst or to perform a needle biopsy of the lump. Being able to see the lesion and the instrument used to withdraw fluid or perform a biopsy increases the accuracy of the procedure. Immediately following the procedure, ultrasound visualization also allows the physician to monitor the area for any changes.

There is no preparation for ultrasound. There is minimal discomfort associated with the test from the pressure of the transducer against the breast, unless it is tender, or if you cannot lie flat without discomfort. You will need to lie on a table undressed from the waist up for the test. The sonographer will apply a gel or oil substance to the breast to improve the transmission of the sound waves. The transducer will be moved over the breast while photographic images are displayed on the video monitor. A radiologist who specializes in reading ultrasound images, or sonograms, will interpret the films. The results of your ultrasound will be sent to the referring physician.

Ultrasound is not recommended by the American College of Radiology as the best method of detecting cancer by screening, but rather as an ancillary procedure after mammography has located an area that needs further evaluation. It is best used to clarify results of a mammogram or when mammography is not suitable because of pregnancy or other reasons.

Breast Cancer Genetic Testing

In 1994 and 1995 two mutated (changed) genes, BRCA1 and BRCA2 (BR=breast, CA=cancer), were discovered that cause 7 - 10 % of breast cancers. A blood test can now determine if a person is a carrier of either mutated gene and the cause of their cancer.

Women who inherit a BRCA1 mutation (changed gene) have a 56 - 80% risk of developing breast cancer by the age of 70 and also up to a 60% chance of developing ovarian cancer. BRCA1 mutations slightly increase the risk for both men and women of developing colon cancer. Women who inherit a BRCA2 mutation also have a 56 - 80% risk of developing breast cancer and a 15 - 20% lifetime chance of developing ovarian cancer. The BRCA2 gene mutation slightly increases the risk for men to have breast cancer as well as prostate cancer. Both gene mutations increase the risk of developing a second primary breast cancer.

After a breast cancer diagnosis, your health care team can review your family and personal history to assess if your cancer is potentially related to a BRCA1 or BRCA2 gene mutation. If you meet the testing criteria, genetic testing can determine if you carry a mutation in either of these identified genes. If positive, your children, male and female, are at a 50% risk of inheriting these defective genes, placing them at higher risk for breast, ovarian or other cancers. Testing consists of having several tablespoons of blood drawn and sent to a laboratory.

Who Is A Candidate For Genetic Testing?

- Person with breast and/or ovarian cancer who has **two or more first* or second-degree*** blood relatives (on one side of family, maternal or paternal) with either breast or ovarian cancer
- Person with breast and/or ovarian cancer who has **one first* or second-degree*** blood relative with breast cancer **younger than 45** (or premenopausal) or a relative who has ovarian cancer **at any age**.
- Personal history of breast and/or ovarian cancer developed **before age 45**
- Personal history of breast and/ or ovarian cancer that is bilateral (both sides) or with multiple primary sites
- Males who develop breast cancer
- Blood relative (first* or second-degree*) of documented BRCA1 or BRCA2 gene carrier
    - ***First-Degree Relatives:** mother, father, sister, brother, daughter, son
    - ***Second-Degree Relatives:** aunt, uncle, grandmother, grandfather, granddaughter, grandson, niece, nephew, half-brother, half-sister

Benefits of BRCA1 and BRCA2 Genetic Testing:

- Allows you to know if your cancer was related to one of these mutated genes
- A negative test might prevent unnecessary anxiety about your children being high risk and prevent future expensive surveillance tests
- Allows family members to choose to be tested or placed in high-risk surveillance programs

Potential Disadvantages of Positive Test Results For Family Members:

- May face discrimination from employers or insurance providers to keep or obtain insurance
- May have emotional or psychological problems knowing they are "high risk" for cancer
- Family members may react unpredictably to positive test results

Appendix B

Understanding Chemotherapy Drugs

There are many drugs used to treat breast cancer. The drugs listed below are the most common. Your physician and nursing staff will be providing you with the names and side-effects of the drugs you will receive.

Chemotherapy drugs are often given in combination. There are many combinations used to treat breast cancer. Your treatment team may refer to the combination of drugs by the initials of each drug. The most common combinations are:

- **CMF**   (Cytoxan, Methotrexate, 5-FU)
- **CAF**   (Cytoxan, Adriamycin, 5-FU)
- **CMFVP** (Cytoxan, Methotrexate, 5-FU, Vincristine, Prednisone)
- **CFP**   (Cytoxan, 5-FU, Prednisone)
- **FAC**   (5-FU, Adriamycin, Cytoxan)

Your treatment team may also refer to the way drugs are given by initials.

- **P.O.** means given by mouth.
- **I.M.** means given by injection into a muscle.
- **S.Q. or S.C.** means given by injection into the fatty (subcutaneous) tissues of body.
- **I.V.** means given by a needle into a vein.

Menstrual Cycle Changes

Chemotherapy drugs may cause your menstrual period to become irregular or stop completely (amenorrhea), affecting your present and future fertility. Your age, type of drugs and length of treatment are influential factors. Cyclophosphamide has the highest influence on causing fertility not to return after treatment. Average percentages of menstrual periods that stop while undergoing combination drug treatment are:

Amenorrhea (no menstrual period) during and months after treatment:

Under 35 years	53%
35- 44 years	84%
45 years and up	94%

Permanent amenorrhea in previously affected women:

under 40 years	86%
40 years and up	96%

121

Cyclophosphamide

Name Brands: Cytoxan and Neosar
Methods Administered: P.O., I.V.
Side Effects: Lowered blood counts (WBCs, Platelets, RBCs), nausea, vomiting, loss of appetite, hair loss, stops menstrual periods, skin darkening
Notify Physician of These Side Effects: Blood in urine, fever, chills, painful urination or unusual bleeding or bruising
Precautions: Drink lots of fluids while taking medication. One to two quarts a day is recommended during the 24-hour period following administration. If the drug is given by mouth, take in the morning and follow with adequate fluids during day.

Doxorubicin

Name Brands: Adriamycin PFS, Adriamycin RDF, ADR
Method Administered: I.V.
Side Effects: Hair loss, sore mouth, nausea, vomiting, lowered blood counts (WBCs, Platelets), changes in heart rhythm, darkening of nailbeds, red urine, painful urination, flu-like symptoms, sensitivity to sun or inflammation of eyes
Notify Physician of These Side Effects: Fast or irregular heartbeat, fever, chills, redness or pain at injection site, shortness of breath, swelling of feet and lower legs, diarrhea for over 24 hours, unusual bleeding or bruising, wheezing, joint pain, side or stomach pain, skin rash or itching, sores in mouth
Precautions: Causes **urine to turn reddish** in color hours after administration, which may stain clothing. This is **not** blood and will last for one to two days after administration. When drug is being administered, if burning or pain occurs at site or in nearby veins, notify your nurse.

Fluorouracil

Name Brands: Adrucil and 5-FU
Method Administered: I.V.
Side Effects: Lowered blood counts (WBCs, Platelets), sore mouth, nausea, vomiting, diarrhea, loss of appetite, some hair loss, sore throat, sensitivity to sunlight, darkening of skin, nail changes, dermatitis or rash, dark veins where drug was administered
Notify Physician of These Side Effects: Chest pain, cough, difficulty with balance, shortness of breath, black tarry stools, diarrhea over 24 hours in duration, fever, chills, sores in mouth, stomach cramps, unusual bleeding or bruising
Precautions: Avoid people with colds and infections. Avoid prolonged exposure to sunlight.

Methotrexate

Name Brand: Folex PFS
Methods Administered: P.O., I.M., I.V.
Side Effects: Sore mouth, nausea, vomiting, loss of appetite, diarrhea, hair loss, taste alterations, blurred vision, dizziness, fatigue, infertility, itching, sensitivity to sun
Notify Physician of These Side Effects: Black tarry stools, bloody vomit, diarrhea over 24 hours in duration, fever, chills, sore throat, sores in mouth, stomach pain or unusual bleeding or bruising
Precautions: Do not drink alcohol while receiving the drug. Avoid too much sun and use of sun lamps or tanning beds. Do not take aspirin or ibuprofen without first checking with your physician.

Paclitaxel

Brand Name: TAXOL
Method of Administration: I.V.
Administration Side Effects: Rare allergic reaction during administration. Nurse will monitor blood pressure, temperature and respirations during infusion. Report immediately: shortness of breath, wheezing, dizziness or light-headedness, sudden onset of nausea, constricted feeling in throat, increase or decrease in heart rate or pain at injection site.
Expected side effects:
Hair loss (occurs from 14 to 21 days after first treatment and includes: scalp, eyebrows, eyelashes and pubic hair). Lowered white blood cells. Muscle and joint pain several days after treatment. Tingling or burning sensation in hands and/or feet
Side effects that should be reported to physician <u>immediately</u>:
Pain, redness or swelling at the injection site while receiving or after the drug has been given. Temperature over 100.5°F. Chills. Blood in urine, stool, vomit or a nosebleed not controlled in 15 minutes. Shortness of breath or wheezing.
Side effect that should be reported <u>within 24 hours</u>:
Vomiting or diarrhea not controlled in 24 hours. Sore throat. Blisters on mouth. Sores in mouth. Painful or frequent urination. Dizziness. Any sore that does not heal or that has signs of infection (pus, redness, swelling)

Vincristine

Brand Names: Oncovin and Vincasar PFS
Method Administered: I.V.
Side Effects: Hair loss, numbness in limbs, nausea, vomiting, lowered blood counts (WBCs and Platelets), ovary suppression, constipation
Notify Physician of These Side Effects: Fever, chills, unusual bleeding or bruising, blurred or double vision, confusion, constipation, difficulty walking, tingling in fingers and toes, sores in mouth, pain in stomach
Precautions: This medication can cause severe constipation. Eat lots of fiber, drink lots of water, and ask your physician about using a stool softener or laxative.

Other Medications

Dexamethasone

Brand Names: Decardon, Dexasone, Dexone, Hexadrol
Methods of Administration: P.O., I.M., I.V.
Side Effects: Euphoria, restlessness, insomnia, stomach irritation, increased appetite
Notify Physician of These Side Effects: Dizziness, fainting, shortness of breath, fever, wounds that don't heal, swelling of feet or legs
Precautions: Take medication with food. Do not take more medication than prescribed. **Do not stop taking medication without informing your physician.**

Prednisone

Brand Names: Deltasone, Liquid Pred, Meticorten, Orasone, Panasol and Prednicen-M.
Method Administered: P.O.
Side Effects: Increase in appetite, indigestion, nervousness or restlessness, trouble in sleeping, sense of well-being, nausea, vomiting, fluid retention
Notify Physician of These Side Effects: Blurred vision, frequent urination, hallucinations, hives or skin rash, abdominal pain or burning, black tarry stools, irregular heart beats, unusual bruising, wounds that do not heal, nausea or vomiting for over 24 hours in duration
Precautions: Take medication at same time of day starting early in morning. Do not take at night or late in afternoon. Do not increase or decrease dose without physician's consent. **Do not stop taking medication without notifying your physician.**

Tamoxifen

Brand Names: Nolvadex, TAM
Method of Administration: P.O.
Side Effects: Hot flashes, nausea when first begun, fluid retention, vaginal discharge, menstrual irregularities, vaginal dryness, may have flare of bone pain when drug is first started (first few weeks of treatment), increase in fertility
Notify Physician of These Side Effects: Excessive vaginal dryness, vaginal infection, changes in vision, continued bone pain
Precautions: Take medication with food. Ask your physician about the need for birth control. A yearly gynecological exam is recommended.

❧ ❧ ❧

Appendix C

Resources

One of the most important ways to gain control over your disease and reduce your anxiety is to get answers to questions you have. Because you are an individual, your questions and needs may be different from other women and not be addressed by your healthcare team. This is when you can reach out to support resources available, most free of charge, and find out what you need to know. Start a notebook for keeping information about your disease, treatment and recovery. Remove the tear-out pages in the back of this book and place them in your notebook. Write down your questions and then read through this list of resources for breast cancer patients. Call or write the resource. In your notebook record your questions, the telephone number, when you called, and who you talked to. Ask them to mail you information and file it in your recovery notebook for future reference.

The Internet is a valuable resource, but be sure that the site you visit is recognized as having sound clinical information. Most national cancer organizations have sites, as well as medical schools and universities. Internet access is available at most public and hospital libraries. A directory of sites is located at: http://www.cancerlinks.org/breastcanlinks.html. Medication side-effects are available from your local pharmacist. Ask your healthcare team for names of local sources of support or call your local hospital library.

American Cancer Society (ACS)
800-ACS-2345
National Office
1599 Clifton Road NE
Atlanta, GA 30329
http://www.cancer.org/bcn.html
Check Yellow Pages for local office address and telephone number.
Provides free, written information on breast cancer, support group information and referral to "Reach to Recovery" program.

National Breast Cancer Coalition
202-296-7477 or 202-265-6854 Fax
1707 L Street NW, Suite 1060
Washington, DC 20036
A grassroots advocacy movement of more than 300 member organizations and thousands of individuals working through a National Action Network, dedicated to the eradication of breast cancer through action, policy and advocacy.

National Cancer Institute (NCI)
800-4 CANCER
Public Inquiry Section, Office of Cancer Communications
Building 31, Room 10 A 24
Bethesda, MD 20892
http://www.nci.nih.gov
Provides free, written information on all aspects of breast cancer

National Alliance of Breast Cancer Organizations (NABCO)
800-719-9154 or 212-889-0606
9 East 37th Street, 10th Floor
New York, NY 10016
http://www.nabco.org/
A non-profit national organization which acts as an advocate for breast cancer patients. Provides information on resources throughout the United States for patients concerning all aspects of breast cancer treatment and recovery. Breast cancer treatment centers list available on request.

Komen Alliance (Susan G. Komen Foundation)
800-I'M AWARE
Occidental Tower
5005 LBJ Freeway, Suite 370
Dallas, Texas 75244
http://www.komen.com/
Offers information on all areas of breast cancer treatment and support.

Y-ME National Breast Cancer Organization
1-800-221-2141 (24 Hour Hotline)
212 W. Van Buren
Chicago, IL 60607
http://www.y-me.org/
Provides support and counseling through a 24-hour hotline. Trained volunteers, all of whom have had breast cancer, are matched by background and experience to callers whenever possible. Information on local support programs in your area or how to establish a support program is available. Referrals for major cancer treatment centers available.

AMC Cancer Research Center's Cancer Information Line
800-525-3777
Professional cancer counselors provide answers to questions about cancer, support and information on free publications. Equipped for deaf and hearing-impaired callers.

Specific Resources

Breast Reconstruction

◆ *The Breast Reconstruction Series* is a free series of fact sheets on breast reconstruction, offered by the National Alliance of Breast Cancer Organizations. Call 212-889-0606.

Exercise

◆ Check with your local YWCA for its special exercise programs for breast cancer survivors called **Encore**. Call YWCA National Headquarters at 212-614-2827 to locate programs in your area.

◆ *In Touch For Life* (Zeneca Pharmaceuticals, 1994) is a free video wellness program with exercise instructions for lumpectomy or mastectomy patients. To order, write to Zeneca/Nolvadex Fulfillment, P. O. Box 15437, Wilmington, DE 19850-15437, or call 800-456-5678 and ask for extension 8609.

◆ **Reach To Recovery**, a program of the American Cancer Society, offers visits from volunteers. Call your local ACS unit for an appointment. Volunteers will share helpful information for recovery, including range of motion exercises for the surgical arm.

Hair Care and Make-Up

◆ **Look Good, Feel Better** is a program of the American Cancer Society which offers free class instructions on makeup application and hair care during cancer treatment. Call your local ACS office or 800-ACS-2345.

◆ *Looking Up: A Complete Guide to Looking and Feeling Good for the Recovering Cancer Patient* is a book by Suzy Kalter (McGraw Hill Book Company, 1987) which offers makeup, hair and grooming tips for patients undergoing cancer treatment. Check your local library or book store.

Insurance or Legal Matters

◆ **The National Insurance Consumer Helpline** is a hotline established to answer consumer questions and provide problem-solving support and printed materials for patients. The lines are manned by trained personnel and licensed agents. The service is available 8:00 a.m. to 8:00 p.m. Eastern Standard Time, Monday through Friday. Call 800-942-4242.

◆ **The National Insurance Consumer Organization** was organized to educate consumers about their insurance rights through publications and telephone inquiries. Call 202-547-6426. Fax 202-547-6427.

◆ *Cancer: Your Job, Insurance and the Law* (4585-PS) is a publication of the American Cancer Society which summarizes cancer patients' legal rights regarding insurance and employment and includes complaint procedure instructions. Call 800-ACS-2345.

◆ *The Americans With Disabilities Act: Protection for Cancer Patients Against Employment Discrimination* (4585, 1993) is an American Cancer Society brochure which defines the ADA law by describing employment rights of the cancer patient. Call 800-ACS-2345.

◆ *The Consumer's Guide To Health Insurance* (C103), *The Consumer's Guide To Long-Term Care Insurance* (C101) and *The Consumer's Guide to Medicare Supplement Insurance* (C101) are guides prepared to help the patient understand health insurance coverage. Call 800-942-4242.

Living Wills

◆ **Choice in Dying** advocates the recognition and protection of individual rights at the end of life and provides counseling for individuals regarding preparing and using advance directives and durable powers of attorney for health care. Write to 200 Varick Street, 10th Floor, Room 1001, New York, NY 10014-4810. Call 800-989-WILL.

Lymphedema

◆ **The North American Vodder Association of Lymphatic Therapy** (NAVALT®) can provide more information on lymphedema and its treatments. Call 1-888-462-8258 (toll free) or 972-243-5959 or 216-729-3258.

◆ For more information on lymphedema and its treatments, contact **The National Lymphedema Network** at (800) 541-3259.

Nutrition
- ◆ **The American Institute for Cancer Research** (AICR) supports research and provides public education exclusively in the area of diet, nutrition and cancer and offers free resources. Call 800-843-8114 or write to 1759 R Street NW, Washington, DC 20069.

Prosthesis
- ◆ Check in the yellow pages of your telephone book. Call your local unit of the American Cancer Society. Ask your surgeon or nurse for references.

- ◆ Y-ME maintains a prosthesis and wig bank for women who cannot afford to purchase one. Call 800-221-2141. If the appropriate size of prosthesis or color of wig is available, it will be mailed anywhere in the country to you for a small shipping fee.

Support Groups
- ◆ Ask your treatment team for the names of local groups. Call the local American Cancer Society office or 800-ACS-2345. Call NABCO 212-889-0606. Call Y-ME at 800-221-2141.

Cancer Treatment Database
- ◆ The National Cancer Institute maintains a cancer treatment database providing prognostic, stage and treatment information on more than 1,000 protocol (treatment) summaries. A computer modem is needed for access to this Physician Data Query (PDQ). For more information, call NCI at 310-496-7403.

*As Survivors,
we know that reading is to the mind
what exercise is to the body. We ensure our
mental health through the wisdom
of others found in books. We read to
learn and grow from others' experiences.*

Appendix D

Recommended Reading

Cancervive: The Challenge of Life After Cancer
Susan Nessim and Judith Ellis
Houghton Mifflin, 1991
Cancer survivors share ways to cope.

Dr. Susan Love's Breast Book
Susan Love, MD, Breast Surgeon
Addison Wesley Publishing, 1991
General reference.

Every Woman's Guide To Breast Cancer
Vickie L. Seltzer, MD
Penguin Viking, 1989
Prevention, treatment and recovery.

Helping Your Mate Face Breast Cancer
Judy C. Kneece, RN, OCN
EduCare Publishing, 1995
Tips on how to become an effective support partner during the breast cancer experience.

Invisible Scars
Mimi Greenberg, Ph.D.
Walker and Company, 1988
A guide to coping with the emotional impact of breast cancer.

Spinning Straw Into Gold: Your Emotional Recovery From Breast Cancer
Kaye, Ronnie, MFCC
Simon & Schuster, 1991
Emotional recovery from breast cancer

The Breast Cancer Companion
Kathy LaTour
William Morrow and Company, 1993
A guide for decisions from diagnosis through recovery.

The Cancer Conqueror
The Triumphant Patient
Greg Anderson
Thomas Nelson, 1992
Two books on how to become an exceptional patient during a cancer diagnosis.

The Race Is Run One Step At A Time: My Personal Struggle And Every Woman's Guide To Taking Charge of Breast Cancer
Nancy Brinker
Simon & Schuster, 1990
Strategies for treatment and recovery.

Continued on next page:

Recommended Reading

Breast Cancer? Let Me Check My Schedule!
Carol Cederberg, Daria Davidson, Joy Edwards, Carol Hebestreit, Betsy Lambert, Amy Langer, Cathy Masamitsu, Sally Snodgrass, Carol Stack, Carol Washington
Innovative Medical Education Consortium, Inc. 1994
Ten professional women tell how they met the challenge of fitting breast cancer into their busy lives

How To Help Children Through A Parent's Serious Illness
Kathleen McCue
St. Martin's Griffin, 1994
ISBN 0-312-146196
Tips on how to help children during the family cancer experience

After Cancer: A Guide To Your New Life
Wendy Schlessel Harpham, MD
Harper Perennial, 1995
ISBN 0-06-097678-0
How to deal with the problems of survivorship after cancer treatment

A Medical and Spiritual Guide to Living With Cancer
William A. Fintel, MD and Gerald R. McDermott, Ph.D.
Word Publishing, 1993
ISBN 0-8499-3504-0
Choosing the right therapy, finding renewed spiritual strength, increasing changes for full recovery

The Wellness Community: Guide to Fighting for Recovery from Cancer
Harold H Benjamin, Ph.D.
G. P. Putnam's Sons, 1994
ISBN: 0-87477-794-1
Recovery guide for patients using a mind/body approach to maximize the effect of the immune system in combination with traditional medicine

What To Do If You Get Breast Cancer
Lydia Komarnicky, MD and Anne Rosenbery, MD
Little, Brown and Company, 1995
ISBN: 0-316-09289-4
Guide to help patients make informed decisions

A Woman's Decision
Karen Berger and John Bostwick III, MD
C. B. Mosby Company, 1984
ISBN 0-345-32485-4
Breast reconstruction decisions

Timeless Healing: The Power and Biology of Belief
Herbert Benson, MD
Fireside, 1997
ISBN 0-684-81441-2
Practical help in conquering illness

Ask your treatment team for their list of recommended reading. You can conduct your own book search on the Internet at: http://www.amazon.com Type in "breast cancer" to find additional topics.

🐦 🐦 🐦

References

Arnold, Elizabeth and Kathleen Boggs. *Interpersonal Relationships.* Philadelphia: W.B. Saunders, 1995.

Bellerson, Karen J. *The Complete & Up-To-Date Fat Book.* Garden City Park, NY: Avery Publishing Group, 1993.

Bland, Kirby I. *The Breast.* Philadelphia, PA: W.B. Saunders, 1998.

Bohmert, Heinz H., and Henry Patrick Leis, Jr. *Breast Cancer.* New York, NY: Thieme Medical Publisher, 1989.

Groenwald, S.L. *Cancer Nursing.* Boston: Jones and Bartlett, 1997

Groenwald, S.L. *Psychosocial Dimensions of Cancer.* Boston: Jones and Bartlett, 1992.

Haagensen, C. D. *Diseases of the Breast.* Philadelphia, PA: W.B. Saunders, 1986.

Harris, Jay R. *Breast Diseases.* Philadelphia: J.B. Lippincott, 1995.

Holland, J. and J. Rowland. *Handbook of Psychooncology.* New York: Oxford University Press, l991.

Lippman, Marc E. *Diagnosis and Management of Breast Cancer.* Philadelphia: W.B. Saunders, 1988.
National Cancer Institute. *Mastectomy.* U.S. Department of Health and Human Affairs, Public Health Service, National Institutes of Health, 1990.

National Cancer Institute. SEER Data. U.S. Department of Health and Human Affairs, Public Health Service, National Institutes of Health, 1990-1991.

National Cancer Institute. *Taking Time.* U. S. Department of Health and Human Affairs, Public Health Service, National Institutes of Health, 1990.

Nessim, S. and Judith Ellis. *Cancervive.* New York: Houghton Mifflin, 1991.

Penneypacker, H. S. *MammaCare Method of Breast Self-Exam.* Gainesville, Florida: MammaTech Corporation.

Pagana, K. and T. Pagana. *Diagnostic Testing and Nursing Implications.* St. Louis, MO: C.V. Mosby, 1990.

Tenenbaum, L. *Cancer Chemotherapy and Biotherapy.* Philadelphia: W.B. Saunders, 1994.

Glossary

It is important to understand the medical terminology related to your diagnosis and treatments. The following is a list of the most common medical terms used in breast cancer. If you do not understand the technical language used by your doctor or nurse, ask them to explain what they mean. Understanding the terms will enable you to make intelligent decisions.

"Ask questions. Be informed. Live one day at a time."
~ Judy M. Sheeks, Survivor

Abscess — A collection of pus from infection.

Acini — The parts of the breast gland where fluid or milk is produced (singular: acinus).

Acute — Occurring suddenly or over a short period of time.

Adenocarcinoma — A form of cancer that involves cells from the lining of the walls of many different organs of the body. Breast cancer is a type of adenocarcinoma.

Adjuvant Treatment — Treatment that is added to increase the effectiveness of a primary treatment. In cancer, adjuvant treatment usually refers to chemotherapy, hormonal therapy or radiation therapy after surgery to increase the likelihood of killing all cancer cells.

Alkylating Agents — Type of chemotherapy drug used in cancer treatment.

Alopecia — Refers to hair loss as a result of chemotherapy or radiation therapy administered to the head. Hair loss from chemotherapy is temporary. Hair loss from radiation is usually permanent.

Amenorrhea — The absence or discontinuation of menstrual periods.

Analgesic — Medicine given to control pain; for example: Aspirin or Tylenol®.

Anesthesia — Medication that causes entire or partial loss of feeling or sensation.

135

Androgen — A male sex hormone. Androgens may be used in patients with breast cancer to treat recurrence of the disease.

Aneuploid — The characteristic of having either fewer or more than the normal number of chromosomes in a cell. This is an abnormal cell.

Anorexia — Severe, uncontrolled loss of appetite.

Antiemetic — A medicine that prevents or relieves nausea and vomiting, used during and sometimes after chemotherapy.

Antimetabolites — Anticancer drugs that interfere with the processes of DNA production, thus preventing cell division.

Areola — The circular field of dark colored skin surrounding the nipple.

Aspiration — Removing fluid or cells from tissue by inserting a needle into an area and drawing the fluid into the syringe.

Asymptomatic — Without obvious signs or symptoms of disease. Cancer may cause symptoms and warning signs; but, especially in its early stages, cancer may develop and grow without producing any symptoms.

Atypical Cells — Not usual; abnormal. Cancer is the result of atypical cell division.

Autologous — Coming from the same person.

Axilla — The armpit.

Axillary Dissection — Surgical removal of lymph nodes from the armpit. This tissue is then sent to the pathologist to determine if the breast cancer has spread outside of the breast. The number of nodes dissected varies during surgery. Your physician can tell you how many nodes were removed.

Axillary Nodes — The lymph nodes in the axilla (underarm) that are cut out and examined during surgery to see if the cancer has spread past the breast. The number of nodes in this area varies.

> **"Absolutely** *nothing in my life prepared me for cancer — except God."*
> ~ Kay C. Harvey, Survivor

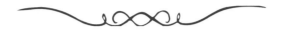

Benign Tumor — An abnormal growth that is not cancer and does not spread to other parts of the body.

Bilateral — Pertains to both sides of the body. For example, bilateral breast cancer would be on both sides of the body or in two breasts.

Biological Response Modifier — Treatment used which alters the body's natural response to stimulate bone marrow to make specific blood cells. Referred to as colony stimulating factors.

Biopsy — The surgical removal of a small piece of tissue or a small tumor for microscopic examination to determine if cancer cells are present. A biopsy is the most important procedure in diagnosing cancer.

Biotherapy — Treatments used to stimulate the body's immune system.

Blood Count — A test to measure the number of red blood cells (RBCs), white blood cells (WBCs) and platelets in a blood sample.

Bone Marrow — The soft, fatty substance filling the cavities of the bones. Blood cells are manufactured in the bone marrow. Chemotherapy will affect the bone marrow, resulting in a temporary decrease in the number of cells in the blood.

Bone Marrow Biopsy and Aspiration — A procedure in which a needle is inserted into the center of a bone, usually the hip, to remove a small amount of bone marrow for microscopic examination.

Bone Scan — The injection of a trace amount of radioactive substance into the bloodstream to illuminate the bones under a special camera to see if the cancer has spread to the bones.

Breast Cancer — If not removed from the body, a potentially fatal tumor because of its ability to leave the breast and go to other vital organs and continue to grow. These are uncontrolled breast cells that are abnormal with uncontrolled growth.

*"... **breast** cancer prompts a desire to take action."*
~ Judy E. Windsor,
Survivor

Breast Implant — A round or teardrop shaped sac inserted into the body to restore the shape of the breast. May be filled with saline water or synthetic material.

Breast Self-Exam (BSE) — A procedure to examine the breasts thoroughly once a month to detect any changes or suspicious lumps. Exams should be practiced at the end of the period or seven days after the start of the period and be performed monthly at the same time.

"Cancer has given me a purpose. It has most assuredly opened both my eyes and my heart."
~ Rose-Marie Bowman Gann, Survivor

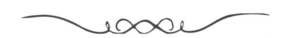

Calcifications — Small calcium deposits in breast tissue seen on mammography. The smallest object detected on mammography. Deposits are the result of cell death. Occurs with benign and malignant changes.

Cancer — A general term used to describe more than 100 different uncontrolled growths of abnormal cells in the body. Cancer cells have the ability to continue to grow, invade and destroy surrounding tissue, leave the original site and travel via lymph or blood systems to other parts of the body where they can set up new cancerous tumors.

Cancer Cell — A cell that divides and reproduces abnormally with uncontrolled growth. This cell can break away and travel to other parts of the body and set up another site, referred to as metastasis.

Clavicle — The collarbone.

Carcinoembryonic Antigen (CEA) — Blood test used to follow women with metastatic breast cancer to help determine if the treatment is working. This is not a test specific for cancer.

Carcinogen — Any substance that initiates or promotes the development of cancer. For example, asbestos is a proven carcinogen.

Carcinoma — A form of cancer that develops in tissues covering or lining organs of the body, such as the skin, the uterus, the lung or the breast.

Carcinoma In Situ — An early stage of development, when the cancer is still confined to the tissues of origin. It has not spread outside the area. In situ carcinomas are highly curable.

CAT Scan or CT Scan — An x-ray view of the body in sections.

Cell — The basic structural unit of all life. All living matter is composed of cells.

Cellulitis — Infection occurring in soft tissues. Your surgical arm has an increased risk for cellulitis because of the removal of lymph nodes. Pain, swelling and warmth occur in the area.

Chemotherapy — Treatment of cancer by use of chemicals. Usually refers to drugs used to treat cancer.

Clinical Trial — Entering into a cancer treatment program that has proven to be effective after experiments. Evidence has proven potential effectiveness, and preliminary studies in humans suggest usefulness.

Combination Chemotherapy — Treatment consisting of the use of two or more chemicals to achieve maximum kill of tumor cells.

Combined Modality Therapy — Two or more types of treatments used to supplement each other. For instance, surgery, radiation, chemotherapy, hormonal or immunotherapy may be used alternatively or together for maximum effectiveness.

Complete Blood Count (CBC) — A laboratory test to determine the number of red blood cells, white blood cells, platelets, hemoglobin and other components of a blood sample.

Computerized Tomography Scans — Commonly called CT or CAT scans. These specialized x-ray studies indicate cancer or metastasis.

Cooper's Ligaments — Flexible bands of tissue that pass from the chest muscle between the lobes of the breasts, providing shape and support the breasts.

Core Biopsy — Removal (with a large needle) of a piece of a lump. The piece is sent to the lab to see if the lump is benign or malignant.

"Cry when you must . . . Remember, it could be worse. Just do your best. Cry and you'll feel better. Dance also if possible."
~ Audrey E. Mitchell, Survivor

139

Cyst — An abnormal saclike structure that contains liquid or semisolid material; is usually benign. Lumps in the breast are often found to be harmless cysts.

Cytology — Study of cells under a microscope that have been sloughed off, cut out or scraped off organs to microscopically examine for signs of cancer.

Cytotoxic — Drugs that can cause the death of cancer cells. Usually refers to drugs used in chemotherapy treatments.

Detection — The discovery of an abnormality in an asymptomatic or symptomatic person.

Diagnosis — The process of identifying a disease by its characteristic signs, symptoms and laboratory findings. With cancer, the earlier the diagnosis is made, the better the chance for cure.

"Don't *withdraw or isolate yourself. Reach out and talk. Spill your emotions . . ."*
~ Kathy Manos, Survivor

Differentiated — The similarity between a normal cell and the cancer cell; defines what degree of change has occurred. Cancer cells that are well differentiated are close to the original cell and are usually less aggressive. Poorly differentiated cells have changed more and are more aggressive.

Diaphanography (DPG) — A non-invasive procedure (no cutting) which uses ordinary light as an investigative tool to detect breast masses. Also called transillumination.

Diploid — The characteristic of having two sets of chromosomes in a cell. This is normal for a breast cell.

DNA — One of two nucleic acids (the other is RNA) found in the nucleus of all cells. DNA contains genetic information on cell growth, division and cell function.

Doubling Time — The time required for a cell to double in number. Breast cancer has been shown to double in size every 23 to 209 days. It would take one cell, doubling every 100 days, eight to ten years to reach one centimeter, 3/8 inch.

Ductal Carcinoma In Situ — A cancer inside the ducts of breast that has not grown through the wall of the duct into the surrounding tissues. Sometimes referred to as a precancer. Good prognosis is involved with in situ cancers.

Ductal Papillomas — Small noncancerous finger-like growths in the mammary ducts that may cause a bloody nipple discharge. Commonly found in women 45 to 50 years of age.

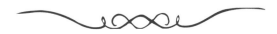

Edema — Excess fluid in the body or a body part that is described as swollen or puffy.

Endocrine Manipulation — Treating breast cancer by changing the hormonal balance of the body to prevent hormone dependent cancer cells from multiplying.

Estrogen — A female hormone secreted by the ovaries which is essential for menstruation, reproduction and the development of secondary sex characteristics, such as breasts. Some patients with breast cancer are given drugs to suppress the production of estrogen in their bodies.

Estrogen Receptor Assay (ERA) — A test that is done on cancerous tissue to see if a breast cancer is hormone-dependent and may be treated with hormonal therapy. The test will reveal if your cancer is estrogen receptor positive or negative.

*"***Even** *though breast cancer totally disrupts your life, it is only a temporary detour"*
~Shelly Belka, Survivor

Excisional Biopsy — Surgical removal of a lump or suspicious tissue by cutting the skin and removing the tissue.

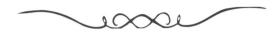

Familial Cancer — One occurring in families more frequently than would be expected by chance.

Fat Necrosis Tumor — Destruction of fat cells in the breast due to trauma or injury that can cause a hard noncancerous lump.

Fibroadenoma — A noncancerous, solid tumor most commonly found in younger women.

Fibrocystic Breast Changes or Condition — A noncancerous breast condition in which multiple cysts or lumpy areas develop in one or both breasts. It can be accompanied by discomfort or pain that fluctuates with the menstrual cycle. Large cysts can be treated by aspiration of the fluid they contain.

*"**Finding** the humor in breast cancer has brought me tremendous physical and psychological healing . . ."*
~ Jane Hill,
Survivor

Fine Needle Aspiration — Procedure to remove cells or fluid from tissues using a needle with an empty syringe. Cells or breast fluid is extracted by pulling back on plunger and then is analyzed by a physician.

Flow Cytometry — A test done on cancerous tissues that shows the aggressiveness of the tumor. It shows how many cells are in the dividing stage at one time, commonly referred to as the 'S' phase, and the DNA content of the cancer, referred to as the ploidy. This reveals how rapidly the tumor is growing.

Frozen Section — A technique in which a part of the biopsy tissue is frozen immediately, and a thin slice is then mounted on a microscope slide, enabling a pathologist to analyze it in just a few minutes for a diagnosis.

Frozen Shoulder — Surgical shoulder which has severely restricted range of motion and is painful.

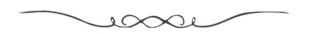

Galactocele — A clogged milk duct, often associated with childbirth.

Genes — Located in the nucleus of the cell, genes contain hereditary information that is transferred from cell to cell.

Genetic — Refers to the inherited pattern located in genes for certain characteristics.

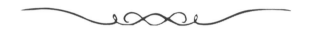

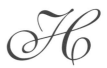

Hematoma — A collection of blood that can form in a wound after surgery, an aspiration or from an injury.

Hormonal Therapy — Treatment of cancer by alteration of the hormonal balance. Some cancer will only grow in the presence of certain hormones.

Hormone — Secreted by various organs in the body, hormones help regulate growth, metabolism and reproduction. Some hormones are used as treatment following surgery for breast, ovarian and prostate cancers.

Hormone Receptor Assay — A diagnostic test to determine whether a breast cancer's growth is influenced by hormones or if it can be treated with hormones.

Hot Flashes — A sensation of heat and flushing that occurs suddenly. May be associated with menopause or some medications.

Hyperplasia — An abnormal excessive growth of cells that is benign.

*"**Humor** helps. Go out each day with joy."*
~ Mildred Hydrick, Survivor

Intramuscular (I.M.) — To receive a medication by needle injection into the muscle of the body.

Immune System — Complex system by which the body protects itself from outside invaders which are harmful to the body.

Immunology — Study of the body's mechanisms of resistance against disease or invasion by foreign substances. The ability of the body to fight a disease.

Immunotherapy — A treatment that stimulates the body's own defense mechanisms to combat diseases such as cancer.

Immunosuppressed — Condition of having a lowered resistance to disease. May be a temporary result of lowered white blood cells from chemotherapy administration.

143

Incisional Biopsy — A surgical incision made through the skin to remove a portion of a suspected lump or tissue.

Inflammation — Reaction of tissue to various conditions which may result in pain, redness or warmth of tissues in the area.

Infiltrating Cancer — Cancer that has grown through the cell wall of the breast area, in which it originated, and into surrounding tissues.

Informed Consent — Process of explanation to the patient of all risks and complications of a procedure or treatment before it is done. Most informed consents are written and signed by the patient or a legal representative.

Intraductal — Residing within the duct of the breast. Intraductal disease may be benign or malignant.

Invasive Cancer — Cancer that has spread outside its site of origin and is growing into the surrounding tissues.

In Situ — In place, localized and confined to one area. A very early stage of cancer.

Infiltrating Ductal Cell Carcinoma — A cancer that begins in the mammary glands and has spread to areas outside the gland.

Intravenous (I.V.) — Entering the body through a vein.

Inverted Nipple — The turning inward of the nipple. Usually a congenital condition; but, if it occurs where it has not previously existed, it can be a sign of breast cancer.

> "**Information** *about my cancer was necessary for me to once again feel in control of my life.*"
> ~Ann Parker, Survivor

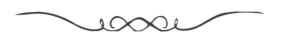

Lactation — Process of being able to produce milk from the breasts.

Lesion — An area of tissue that is diseased.

Leukocyte — A white blood cell or corpuscle.

Leukopenia — A decrease in the number of white blood cells, resulting in susceptibility to infection.

Linear Accelerator — A machine that produces high energy x-ray beams to destroy cancer cells.

Liver Scan — A way of visualizing the liver by injecting into the bloodstream a trace dose of a radioactive substance which helps visualize the organ during x-ray.

Lobular — Pertaining to the part of the breast that is furthest from the nipple, the lobes.

Localized Cancer — A cancer still confined to its site of origin.

Lump — Any kind of abnormal mass in the breast or elsewhere in the body.

Lumpectomy — A surgical procedure in which only the cancerous tumor and an area of surrounding tissue is removed. Usually the surgeon will remove some of the underarm lymph nodes at the same time. This procedure is also referred to as a tylectomy.

Lymphatic Vessels — Vessels that remove cellular waste from the body by filtering through lymph nodes and eventually emptying into the vascular (blood) system.

Lymph — A clear fluid circulating throughout the body in the lymphatic system that contains white blood cells and antibodies.

Lymph Glands — Also called lymph nodes. These are rounded body tissues in the lymphatic system that vary in size from a pinhead to an olive and may appear in groups or one at a time. The principal ones are in the neck, underarm and groin. These glands produce lymphocytes and monocytes (white blood cells which fight foreign substances) and serve as filters to prevent bacteria from entering the bloodstream. They will filter out cancer cells but will also serve as a site for metastatic disease. The major ones serving the breast are in the armpit. Some are located above and below the collarbone and some in between the ribs near the breastbone. There are three levels of lymph nodes in the underarm area of the breast and another around the breast bone. Number of nodes vary from person to person. Lymph nodes are usually sampled

*"**Live** life one day at a time. You can't change yesterday. Forget those '**if only**' thoughts. Worrying about tomorrow only makes things worse."*
~ Harriett Barrineau, Survivor

during surgery to determine if the cancer has spread outside of the breast area.

Lymphedema — A swelling in the arm caused by excess fluid that collects after the lymph nodes have been removed by surgery or affected by radiation treatments.

Macrocyst — A cyst that is large enough to be felt with the fingers.

Magnification View — Special enlarged views to magnify an area for greater detail of suspicious finding. Used in mammography.

Magnetic Resonance Imaging (MRI) — A magnet scan; a form of x-ray using magnets instead of radiation. MRI gives a more clearly defined picture of fatty tissue than x-ray.

Malignant Tumor — A mass of cancer cells. These cells have uncontrolled growth and will invade surrounding tissues and spread to distant sites of the body, setting up new cancer sites, a process called metastasis.

Mammary Duct Ectasia — A noncancerous breast disease most often found in women during menopause. The ducts in or beneath the nipple become clogged with cellular and fatty debris. The duct may have gray to greenish discharge, a lump you can feel and can become inflamed, causing pain.

Mammary Glands — The breast glands that produce and carry milk by way of the mammary ducts to the nipples during pregnancy and breast feeding.

Mammogram — An x-ray of the breast that can detect tumors before they can be felt. A baseline mammogram is performed on healthy breasts usually at the age of 35 to establish a basis for later comparison.

Mammotest — Biopsy (stereotactic) performed under mammography while breast is compressed and lesion is viewed by physician. Sample of lesion is removed using a large core needle and is then sent to lab to determine if it is benign or malignant.

*"**Music** has always been an important part of my life. Whenever I felt the need for a boost, I'd start singing."*
~ Louise K. Edwards, Survivor

Margins — The area of tissue surrounding a tumor when it is removed by surgery.

Mastalgia — Pain occurring in the breast.

Mastectomy — Surgical removal of the breast and some of the surrounding tissue.

> **Modified Radical Mastectomy** — The most common type of mastectomy. Breast skin, nipple, areola and underarm lymph nodes are removed. The chest muscles are saved.

> **Prophylactic Mastectomy** — A procedure sometimes recommended for patients at a very high risk for developing cancer in one or both sides.

> **Subcutaneous Mastectomy** — Performed before cancer is detected, removes the breast tissue but leaves the outer skin, areola and nipple intact. (This is not suitable with a diagnosis of cancer.)

> **Radical Mastectomy (Halsted Radical)** — The surgical removal of the breast, breast skin, nipple, areola, chest muscles and underarm lymph nodes.

> **Segmental Mastectomy (Partial Mastectomy/Lumpectomy)** — A surgical procedure in which only a portion of the breast is removed, including the cancer and the surrounding margin of healthy breast tissue.

Mastitis — Infection occurring in the breast. Pain, tenderness, swelling, redness and warmth may be observed. Usually related to infection and will respond to antibiotic treatment.

Menopause — The time in a woman's life when the menstrual cycle ends and the ovaries produce lower levels of hormones; usually occurs between the age of 45 and 55.

Metastasis — The spread of cancer from one part of the body to another through the lymphatic system or the bloodstream. The cells in the new cancer location are the same type as those in the original sites.

"My mate was excellent in comforting me and letting me know that nothing would change between us."
~ Diane Rice, Survivor

Microcalcifications — Particles observed on a mammogram that are found in the breast tissue, appearing as small spots on the picture. Usually occur from calcium deposits caused by death of breast cells which may be benign or malignant. When clustered in one area, may need to be checked more closely for a malignant change in the breast.

Microcyst — A cyst that is too small to be felt but may be observed on mammography or ultrasound screening.

Micrometastasis — Undetectable spread of cancer outside of the breast that is not seen on routine screening tests. Metastasis is too limited to have created enough mass to be observed.

Multicentric — More than one origin or place of growth in the breast. These growths may or may not be related to each other.

Myleosuppression — A decrease in the ability of the bone marrow cells to produce blood cells, including red blood cells, white blood cells and platelets. This condition increases susceptibility to infection and produces fatigue.

> *"The **medical** bills have been overwhelming . . . but, by the grace of God, I'm trying."*
> ~ Anonymous Survivor

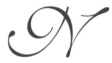

Needle Biopsy — Removal of a sample of tissue from the breast using a wide-core needle with suction.

Necrosis — Death of a tissue.

Neoplasm — Any abnormal growth. Neoplasms may be benign or malignant, but the term usually is used to describe a cancer.

Nodularity — Increased density of breast tissue, most often due to hormonal changes, which cause the breast to feel lumpy in texture. This finding is called normal nodularity, and it usually occurs in both breasts.

Nodule — A small, solid mass.

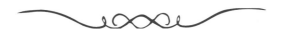

Oncogene — Certain stretches of cellular DNA. Genes that, when inappropriately activated, contribute to the malignant transformation of a cell.

Oncologist — A physician who specializes in cancer treatment.

Oncology — The science dealing with the physical, chemical and biological properties and features of cancer, including causes, the disease process and therapies.

One-Step Procedure — A procedure in which a surgical biopsy is performed under general anesthesia and if cancer is found, a mastectomy or lumpectomy is done immediately as part of the same operation.

Oophorectomy — The surgical removal of the ovaries, sometimes performed as a part of hormone therapy.

Osteoporosis — Softening of bones that occurs with age, calcium loss and hormone depletion.

"Overcoming *fear is the first step to survival."*
~ Lisa Boccard, Survivor

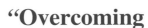

Per Orally (P.O.) — To take a medication by mouth.

Palliative Treatment — Therapy that relieves symptoms, such as pain or pressure, but does not alter the development of the disease. Its primary purpose is to improve the quality of life.

Palpation — A procedure using the hands to examine organs such as the breast. A palpable mass is one you can feel with your hands.

Pathology — The study of disease through the microscopic examination of body tissues and organs. Any tumor suspected of being cancerous must be diagnosed by pathological examination.

Pathologist — A physician with special training in diagnosing diseases from samples of tissue.

Pectoralis Muscles — Muscular tissues attached to the front of the chest wall and extending to the upper arms. These are under the breast. They are divided into the pectoralis major and the pectoralis minor muscles.

Permanent Section — A technique in which a thin slice of biopsy tissue is mounted on a slide to be examined under a microscope by a pathologist in order to establish a diagnosis.

Platelet — A cell formed by the bone marrow and circulating in the blood that is necessary for blood clotting. Platelet transfusions are used in cancer patients to prevent or control bleeding when the number of platelets have decreased.

Ploidy — The number of chromosome sets in a cell.

*"**Put** it all in God's hands and trust Him for the strength you'll need."*
~ Virginia Reid, Survivor

Port, Life Port, Port-A-Cath — A device surgically implanted under the skin, usually on the chest, that enters a large blood vessel and is used to deliver medication, chemotherapy, blood products and also is used to obtain blood samples. A port is usually inserted if a person has veins in the arm which are difficult to use for treatment or if certain types of chemotherapy drugs are to be given.

Precancerous — Abnormal cellular changes that are potentially capable of becoming cancer. These early lesions are very amenable to treatment and cure. Also called pre-malignant.

Progesterone — Female hormone produced by the ovaries during a specific time in the menstrual cycle. Causes the uterus to prepare for pregnancy and the breasts to get ready to produce milk.

Progesterone Receptor Assay (PRA) — A test that is done on cancerous tissue to see if a breast cancer is progesterone hormone dependent and can be treated by hormonal therapy.

Prognosis — A prediction of the course of the disease—the future prospect for the patient. For example, most breast cancer patients who receive treatment early have a good prognosis.

Prolactin — Female hormone which stimulates the development of the breasts and later is essential for starting and continuing milk production.

Prophylactic Mastectomy — Removal of high-risk breast tissue to prevent future development of cancer.

Prosthesis — An artificial form. In the case of breast cancer following mastectomy, a breast form that can be worn inside a bra.

Protocol — A schedule of selected drugs and treatment time intervals known to be effective against a certain cancer.

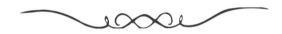

Radiation Therapy — Treatment with high energy x-rays to destroy cancer cells.

Radiation Oncologist — A physician specifically trained in the use of high energy x-rays to treat cancer.

Radiologist — A physician who specializes in diagnoses of diseases by the use of x-rays.

Radiotherapy — Treatment of cancer with high energy radiation. Radiation therapy may be used to reduce the size of a cancer before surgery or to destroy any remaining cancer cells after surgery. Radiotherapy can be helpful in shrinking recurrent cancer to relieve symptoms such as pain and pressure.

Recurrence — Reappearance of cancer after a period of remission.

Regional Involvement — The spread of cancer from its original site to nearby surrounding areas. Regional cancers are confined to one location of the body. Regional involvement in breast cancer could include spread to the lymph nodes or to the chest wall.

Rehabilitation — Programs that help patients adjust and return to full, productive lives. May involve physical therapy, the use of a prosthesis, counseling and emotional support.

*"**Right now**, I'm more assertive. I figured one of the worst things possible has already happened to me, so what have I got to fear?"*
~ MaryAnn Eubanks,
Survivor

*"The **reality** of no breasts made me feel like an 'it.' It was truly silent suffering. Yet, now, I can talk about it, when before, I was mortified."*
~ Anonymous Survivor

Relapse — The reappearance of cancer after a disease-free period.

Remission — Complete or partial disappearance of the signs and symptoms of disease in response to treatment. The period during which a disease is under control. A remission, however, is not necessarily a cure.

Retraction — Process of skin pulling in toward breast tissue, often referred to as dimpling.

Risk Factors — Anything that increases an individual's chance of getting a disease such as cancer. The risk factors for breast disease are a first degree relative with breast cancer, a high fat diet, early menstruation, late menopause, first child after 30 or no children.

Risk Reduction — Techniques used to reduce your chances of getting a certain cancer. For example, reducing your dietary fat may help prevent breast cancer.

S Phase — Test that is performed to determine how many cells within the tumor are in a stage of division.

Sarcoma — A form of cancer that arises in the supportive tissues such as bone, cartilage, fat or muscle.

Secondary Tumor — A tumor that develops as a result of metastasis or spreads beyond the original cancer.

Secondary Site — A second site in which cancer is found. Example: cancer in the lymph nodes near the breast is a secondary site.

Side Effects — Usually describes situations that occur after treatments. For example, hair loss may be a side effect of chemotherapy; fatigue may be a side effect of radiation therapy.

Staging — An evaluation of the extent of the disease, such as breast cancer. A classification based on stage at diagnosis which helps determine the appropriate treatment and prognosis. In breast cancer, it is determined by whether the lymph nodes are involved;

152

whether the cancer has spread to other parts of the body (through the lymphatic system or bloodstream) and set up distant metastasis; and the size of the tumor. Five different stages are used in breast cancer with levels in each stage. Stage IV is the most serious.

Stellate — Appearing on mammography as a star-shape because of the irregular growth of cells into surrounding tissue. May be associated with a malignancy or some benign conditions.

Stereotactic Needle Biopsy — Biopsy done while breast is compressed under mammography. A series of pictures locate the lesion, and a radiologist enters information into a computer. The computer calculates information and positions a needle to remove the finding. A needle is inserted into the lump, and a piece of tissue is removed and sent to the lab for analysis. May be referred to as mammotest or core biopsy.

Stomatitis — Inflammation of the gastrointestinal tract creating discomfort and a potential for infection. May be caused by chemotherapy drugs.

Supraclavicular Nodes — The nodes located above the collar bone in the area of the neck.

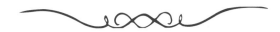

Tamoxifen — An anti-estrogen drug that may be given to women with estrogen receptive tumors to block estrogen from entering the breast tissues. May produce menopause-like symptoms, including hot flashes and vaginal dryness. Currently being used with high risk women in clinical trials to prevent breast cancer and women who have had breast cancer to prevent recurrence.

Thrombocytopenia — A decrease in the number of platelets in the blood, resulting in the potential for increased bleeding and decreased ability for clotting.

Tissue — A collection of similar cells. There are four basic types of tissues in the body: epithelial, connective, muscle and nerve.

"Sharing with other breast cancer patients is very important. You cannot, must not, need not, do it alone!"
~ Felicia Smith, Survivor

"Time *is a healer.***"**
~ Carol C. Criminger,
Survivor

Transillumination — The inspection of an organ by passing a light through the tissues. Transmission of the light varies with different tissue densities.

Tumor — An abnormal tissue, swelling or mass, may be either benign or malignant.

Two-Step Procedure — When surgical biopsy and breast surgery are performed in two separate surgeries.

Ultrasound Examination — The use of high frequency sound waves to locate a tumor inside the body. Helps determine if a breast lump is solid tissue or filled with fluids.

Ultrasound Guided Biopsy — The use of ultrasound to guide a biopsy needle to obtain a sample of tissue for analysis by a pathologist.

*"When I was young, I thought
that a diagnosis of breast cancer
would end the world for me.
Today, at 72, I see things differently.
It's an experience many women share,
and it is not a reason for shame.*
We can be proud that we survive."
~ Carol Hardgrove,
Survivor

Index

Managing My Fears

List all the fears and worries you are presently facing. In the second column list the name of the most appropriate person with whom to verbalize these fears. In the third column think about and list things you can do to change or reduce these fears.

Fear	Person(s) Involved	Things I Can Do

"To fight fear ACT. To increase fear–wait, put off, postpone."
~ David Joseph Schwartz

"You can gain strength, courage, and confidence by every experience in which you really stop to look fear in the face. The danger lies in refusing to face the fear, in not daring to come to grips with it. You must do something you think you cannot do."
~ Eleanor Roosevelt

Managing My Fears

List all the fears and worries you are presently facing. In the second column list the name of the most appropriate person with whom to verbalize these fears. In the third column think about and list things you can do to change or reduce these fears.

Fear	Person(s) Involved	Things I can do

Questions About Surgery

Check the questions you would like to have answered.
Tear out this sheet and take it to your surgical consultation.

Surgeon's Name _____ **Date**_____

General Questions

❑ What is the name of the type of breast cancer I have?

❑ How large was the tumor?

❑ Was the tumor in situ (inside ducts) or invasive (grown through ducts)?

❑ Do you expect the tumor to be found in my lymph nodes?

❑ Do you expect the tumor to have invaded anything else (skin, muscle, bones, other organs)?

❑ Is there any evidence from my mammogram that there might be cancer anywhere else in this breast or in the opposite breast?

❑ Does my type of cancer have an increased incidence of being or occurring in the opposite breast?

Additional Questions _____

_____

_____

Lumpectomy Questions

❑ Am I a candidate for a lumpectomy?

❑ If so, how do you expect my breast to appear after surgery, considering the size of the lump and tissue you need to remove compared to the size of my breast, or the position of the lump in the breast? Do you think it will it be cosmetically acceptable?

❑ Which of the lumpectomy procedures do you plan to use (Segmental, Tylectomy, Lumpectomy)?

❑ Will you remove lymph nodes by a separate incision under my arm?

❑ What do you consider are the advantages and disadvantages of a lumpectomy for my case?

❑ Will a lumpectomy give me the same chance for cure/control of my cancer as a mastectomy?

❑ Will I need to have radiation therapy after a lumpectomy?

❑ How long will I be in the hospital?

❑ Will I have drains in the incision after surgery? Will I go home with drains?

❑ When do you expect the drains to be removed?

❑ How long will I need to be away from my job?

Additional Questions _____

_____

_____

Mastectomy Questions

❑ Which type of mastectomy do you plan to perform?
❑ What do you think are the advantages and disadvantages of my having a mastectomy?
❑ In my particular case, does mastectomy offer a better chance of cure or control of my cancer?
❑ How many and what levels of lymph nodes do you plan to remove?
❑ Will I have drain bulbs in my incision after surgery? If so, how many?
❑ Will I go home with drains in place?
❑ When are drains usually removed?
❑ Will I have to have stitches/sutures removed? When and where will this be done?
❑ How long will I be in the hospital?
❑ When should I be able to resume my normal activities?
❑ Are there any types of limitations which I should expect in my surgical arm in the future?

Additional Questions _____

_____

_____

Reconstruction Questions

❑ Am I a candidate for immediate reconstruction?
❑ Can you provide me with information about immediate reconstruction?
❑ Tell me the advantages of immediate reconstruction. Tell me the disadvantages of immediate reconstruction.
❑ Could you provide me with information on the use of implants and the potential use of my body parts for reconstruction?
❑ Do you foresee anything in my present health status which could prevent me from having either types of reconstruction?

Additional Questions _____

_____

_____

Final Questions

❑ Is there anything else you need to tell me about my cancer or surgery?
❑ Do you have any written information on my cancer or surgery?
❑ Do you recommend any books or videos?
❑ Do you recommend any support group or professional counselor?
❑ If I have additional questions, whom should I call and ask to speak to? (nurse/physician)

Additional Questions _____

_____

_____

Ask your physician to draw where your tumor is located
in your breast and the estimated amount of tissue that will be
removed during surgery.

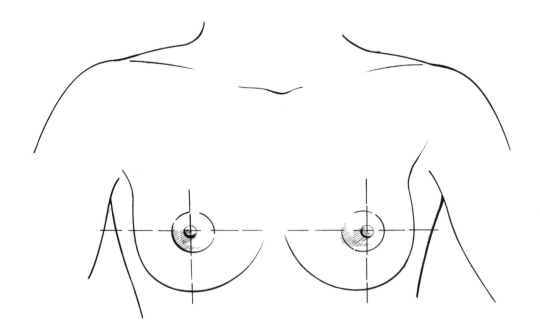

Ask your physician to draw the estimated size of your tumor on this chart.

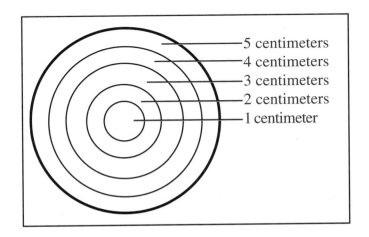

5 centimeters
4 centimeters
3 centimeters
2 centimeters
1 centimeter

Ask your surgeon to draw your planned incision on the back of this page.

Ask your surgeon to draw how your body will look after surgery.

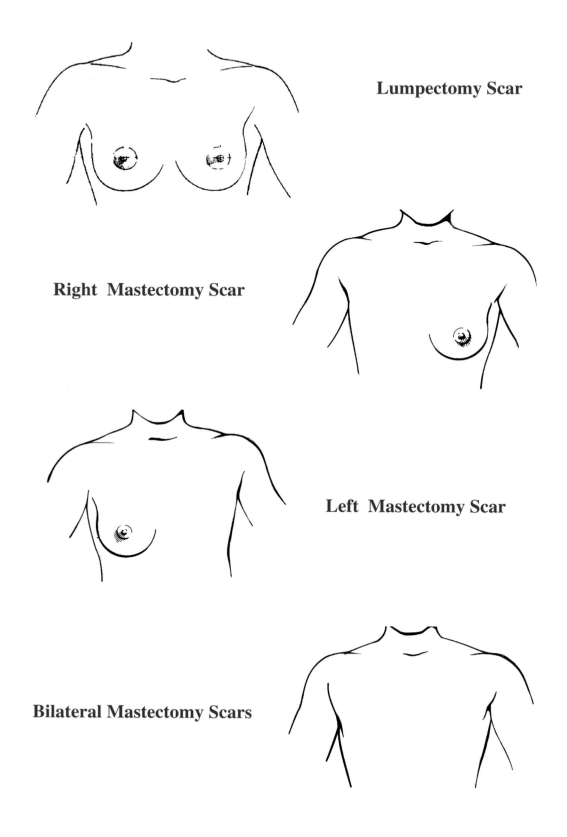

Lumpectomy Scar

Right Mastectomy Scar

Left Mastectomy Scar

Bilateral Mastectomy Scars

Reconstructive Surgeon's Questions

Check the questions you would like to have answered.
Tear out this sheet and take it to your reconstructive consultation.

Surgeon's Name _____   **Date**_____

- ❏ What type of surgery do you recommend for me?
- ❏ Do you suggest use of my own body tissue or an implant?
- ❏ What kind of implants do you recommend? Will they be placed under the muscle?
- ❏ What are the risks and benefits of this surgery?
- ❏ Could I see photographs and talk to some of your patients?
- ❏ What can I expect to look like after surgery?
- ❏ Will you reconstruct my nipple and areola?
- ❏ How much feeling (sensation) will I have in my reconstructed breast?
- ❏ How will my breast feel when touched? (soft, firm)?
- ❏ Will this surgery cause me to have additional scars?
- ❏ How many surgical procedures will my reconstruction require?
- ❏ How long will I be in surgery for each of these procedures?
- ❏ How long will I be in the hospital for each procedure?
- ❏ How often will I need a return appointment with you?
- ❏ How long will it take to complete the reconstruction process?
- ❏ How long before I can return to work or normal activities after each procedure?
- ❏ How much will it cost and how much should my insurance cover?

Additional Questions _____
_____
_____
_____
_____
_____

Breast Reconstructive Surgery Choices

Type and Description	Comments
Tissue Expander An empty silicone sack is implanted under the skin and muscle. It is gradually filled with saline (salt water) solution through a valve over a period of several weeks to stretch the skin before a permanent implant is inserted . General anesthesia is usually used. Outpatient or inpatient. Surgery takes 1 - 2 hours. Second outpatient surgery is required to remove the expander and position the permanent implant and perform nipple and areolar reconstruction. General anesthesia is usually used.	Most common type of reconstructive surgery after breast cancer. May be difficult to match larger opposite breast. Good for bilateral reconstruction. Patient usually returns to physician's office every week for injections of saline into the expander. Injections may cause slight discomfort for the first twenty four hours after filling the expander.
Implant (fixed volume implant) Sack filled with silicone gel or saline fluid is implanted under skin and chest muscle. General anesthesia is used. Outpatient or inpatient surgery: 1 - 2 hours for surgery.	Silicone gel or saline implants can be used. Tissue expanders may be required to stretch the muscle and skin to allow for permanent implant insertion.
Latissimus dorsi (back flap) The back muscle, the latissimus dorsi, along with an eye-shaped wedge of skin are rotated from the back to the breast and sewn in place, leaving the tissues attached to their original blood supply. Inpatient procedure with general anesthesia: 2 - 3 hours surgical time. Flap may be also be used over an implant to give a more natural result, especially to match a larger opposite breast.	Major surgery. Moderately painful. Hospitalization is from 1 - 3 days. Scar left on back. Drains may be left in place for several weeks. May or may not require use of an implant in addition to your own tissue. Some procedures can be performed endoscopically (using special instruments under the skin) that leave smaller scar on the back.
Tram Flap (tummy tuck) The Tram (<u>t</u>ransverse <u>r</u>ectus <u>a</u>bdominous <u>m</u>yocutaneous <u>m</u>uscle) Flap (tummy tuck) One or both rectus muscles (major stomach muscles) are moved up along with fat and skin of lower abdomen and tacked in place to form a breast. Tissue may remain connected to original blood supply, or will require microsurgery. Inpatient surgery with general anesthesia: 3 - 5 hours.	Major surgery and may be painful. Drains in place. Hospitalization is from 3 - 5 days. Difficulty standing up straight for several days or weeks. Scar on abdomen. No implant required is major advantage. 4 - 6 weeks recovery from surgery.
Free Flap (microsurgery) Muscles and fat from other body parts such as buttocks or thighs are detached (cut free) from their blood supply and attached to the breast area blood supply with microsurgery. Surgery can range from 3 to 8 hours according to the degree of reattachment necessary. Inpatient procedure with general anesthesia.	Moderately painful. Uses patient's own tissue. No implant required. Requires surgeon with expertise in microsurgery. Most complex of all reconstructive procedures. Hospitalization from 3 - 5 days. Longest recovery period.
Nipple Reconstruction Nipples are reconstructed from existing skin and fat on the breast. The skin is molded to form the shape of the nipple on the breast mound. Areola reconstruction may also be done. The dark pigmented color is tattooed to match the color of the other areola.	Nipple reconstruction is not major surgery. Pain is usually minimal. Soreness may last for several weeks. Most often done as a second stage procedure following one of the primary reconstructions listed above. Outpatient procedure.

Personal Health Care Directory

Primary Physician _____   **Telephone** _____

Nurse _____   **Address** _____

• •

Surgeon _____   **Telephone** _____

Nurse _____   **Address** _____

• •

Oncologist _____   **Telephone** _____

Nurse _____   **Address** _____

• •

Radiation Oncologist _____   **Telephone** _____

Nurse _____   **Address** _____

• •

Plastic Surgeon _____   **Telephone** _____

Nurse _____   **Address** _____

• •

Others

**Breast Health
Specialist** _____   **Telephone** _____

Pharmacy _____   **Telephone** _____

Hospital _____   **Telephone** _____

_____   **Telephone** _____

Personal Treatment Record

Name _____

Baseline Vital Signs _____

Blood Pressure _____ **Pulse** _____ **Respirations** _____ **Weight** _____

Allergies _____

Routine Medications _____

Date of Diagnosis _____ **Date of Surgery** _____

Diagnosis _____ **Size of Tumor** _____ **Node Status** _____

ER/PR Status _____ **Other Tests** _____

Chemotherapy Drugs _____
_____

Dates of Chemotherapy Treatment
Start _____
_____
_____
Completion _____
_____

Dates of Radiation Therapy
Start _____
_____
_____
Completion _____
_____

Hormonal Therapy _____
_____
_____

Chemotherapy Administration Notes

Radiation Therapy Notes

Bulb Drain Record

Please measure and record drainage of bulb(s) each time you empty drain.

Take this record to your physician.

DATE	TIME	DRAIN 1	DRAIN 2	TOTAL

Bulb Drain Record

Please measure and record drainage of bulb(s) each time you empty drain.

Take this record to your physician.

DATE	TIME	DRAIN 1	DRAIN 2	TOTAL

Hospital Discharge Instructions

Prior to leaving the hospital, your nurse will provide you with verbal and written instructions concerning your care and a list of symptoms that might occur and need to be reported to the doctor. During your hospitalization, it may be helpful to write down any questions as they occur. When your doctor makes the final hospital visit, you may want to be prepared to clarify the following. Check the questions you wish to have answered.

- ☐ If you do not remember what he said about your surgery or diagnosis the day you had surgery, ask him to clarify.
- ☐ What activities can I do with my surgical arm until my next appointment?
- ☐ Are there any special exercises or recommendations regarding the use of my arm?
- ☐ Will the numbness, tingling or sensations experienced be temporary or permanent?
- ☐ What medications will I take for pain?
- ☐ What type of pain is normal after my type of surgery?
- ☐ Will I be given any prescriptions for medication to take home?
- ☐ Do I resume previous medications (especially estrogen-type medications)?
- ☐ When can I shampoo my hair?
- ☐ When can I shower or take a tub bath?
- ☐ When can I remove my bandage?
- ☐ When can I drive?
- ☐ When and how do I make my next appointment?
- ☐ Will I be referred to any other doctors or have any other treatments?
- ☐ If so, when will I see these doctors?
- ☐ When will my pathology report be available?
- ☐ Is there anything special that I can do to ensure a speedy recovery?

Ask your nurse to write down any appointment dates or names of doctors that you will be referred to for further evaluation concerning treatment.

Additional Questions_____
_____
_____

173

Hospital Discharge Instructions Notes

Prosthesis Selection Questions

Check the questions you would like to have answered.
Tear out this sheet and take it with you when searching for a prosthesis.

❑ How do I clean my prosthesis?

❑ Can I get it wet?

❑ How long will it take to dry?

❑ Does perspiration damage the prosthesis?

❑ Will pool chemicals cause any damage?

❑ Is there an exchange policy if I decide it does not meet my needs?

❑ How long should the prosthesis last?

❑ How much will my insurance provider pay toward the cost?

❑ Does my insurance company pay for mastectomy bras?

❑ If yes, how many bras will my insurance pay for at my initial purchase?

❑ How often will my insurance provider pay replacement costs of my prosthesis?

❑ How often will they pay for replacement bras?

❑ Do you bill the provider for the cost, or do I pay and bill my provider?

❑ If I alter them, can I wear my regular bras with the prosthesis I selected?

Additional Questions _____

_____

_____

Prosthesis Selection Notes

Oncologist's Questions

Check the questions you would like to have answered.
Tear out this sheet and take it to your appointment with the oncologist.

Physician's Name _____ **Date**_____

- ❑ What kind of treatment will I receive? (chemotherapy, hormonal, immunotherapy)
- ❑ On what schedule will I receive these treatments?
- ❑ How long will I receive treatments?
- ❑ Where will I receive my treatments? (office, clinic, hospital)
- ❑ Can someone come with me when I receive my treatments?
- ❑ How long will each treatment take?
- ❑ Will I feel like driving myself home after my treatment or do I need a driver?
- ❑ What are the names of the drugs?
- ❑ Are they given by mouth or into a vein?
- ❑ Will I need a port (device implanted under the skin) to receive any I.V. medications or will you use a vein in my arm?
- ❑ What side effects will I experience from the treatments? (nausea, hair loss, changes in blood cell counts, etc.)
- ❑ Will I be given medications to treat side effects?
- ❑ Should I eat before I come for my treatments?
- ❑ Can I take vitamins or herbs if I so choose?
- ❑ What kind of protective precautions to my skin should I take during chemotherapy? (exposure to sunlight)
- ❑ Will any other tests be given before or while I receive my chemotherapy?
- ❑ Will I continue to have my menstrual periods? If not, when will they return?
- ❑ Should I use birth control? What type do you recommend?
- ❑ Will I be able to conceive and bear a child after treatments?
- ❑ What physical changes should I report to you or to your nurse during treatment?
- ❑ Will I need radiation therapy?
- ❑ Can I continue my usual work or exercise schedules, or will I need to modify them during treatments?
- ❑ Are there any precautions my family should take to limit exposure to the chemotherapy during my treatments? (shared eating utensils, bathroom facilities)
- ❑ How will you evaluate the effectiveness of the treatments?
- ❑ When I complete my treatments, how often will I return for checkups?
- ❑ Do you have written information on my cancer or treatment plans?

Additional Questions _____

_____

Oncology Consultation Notes

Radiation Oncologist's Questions

Check the questions you would like to have answered.
Tear out this sheet and take it with you to your radiation consultation.

Physician's Name _____ **Date**_____

❑   How many radiation treatments will I receive?

❑   How long will my first visit take to mark the area?

❑   How do you mark the area that will be radiated?

❑   What kind of soap and bath do you recommend during the treatments?

❑   Is there anything that I cannot use during my treatment? (deodorant, perfume, lotions
      to the chest or back, etc.)

❑   Can I wear a bra or my prosthesis?

❑   Do you have written information on radiation therapy for the breast area?

❑   What side effects are considered normal during therapy?

❑   What side effects, if they occur, should I report immediately?

Additional Questions _____
_____
_____
_____
_____
_____
_____
_____
_____
_____

Radiation Oncology Consultation Notes

Patient Appointment Worksheet

What I Need to Ask or Tell My Health Care Team

Next scheduled appointment: _____

Physician _____ **Date** _____ **Time** _____

Questions to Ask Physician

◆ _____
◆ _____
◆ _____
◆ _____

Questions to Ask Nurse

◆ _____
◆ _____
◆ _____
◆ _____

Remember to Tell Physician/Nurse

◆ _____
◆ _____
◆ _____

It is helpful to write down questions for your nurse or physician prior to your visit and have them answered. It is also helpful to keep a list of items which need to be relayed to your health care team.

181

Patient Appointment Worksheet

What I Need to Ask or Tell My Health Care Team

Next scheduled appointment:

Physician _____ **Date** _____ **Time** _____

Questions to Ask Physician

◆ _____

◆ _____

◆ _____

◆ _____

Questions to Ask Nurse

◆ _____

◆ _____

◆ _____

◆ _____

Remember to Tell Physician/Nurse

◆ _____

◆ _____

◆ _____

It is helpful to write down questions for your nurse or physician prior to your visit and have them answered. It is also helpful to keep a list of items which need to be relayed to your health care team.

Exercise Guidelines After Breast Cancer

Name: _____

Physician: _____

Date: _____

It is proven that a regular program of walking during breast cancer treatment can significantly increase the quality of life for a patient. However, it is important to get your physician's approval before starting this or any exercise program.

Recommended Walking Exercise Program:

Frequency: 4 times a week minimum, 6 times a week maximum; try not to skip more than 1 day in a row if your health allows

Goal: Gradually increase and maintain your heart rate at 100 - 120 beats/minute during walking

Duration: Brisk walking at your own rate; starting at 10 minutes per session and increasing gradually to 30 minutes per session as tolerated

Place: Outdoors preferably when weather permits, indoor mall or treadmill

Attire: Comfortable shoes designed for walking; layered, loose, cotton clothing to absorb perspiration; and personal identification in case of an emergency

Recommended Routine:

1. 5 minutes slow walking to warm-up
2. Increase walking to a brisk pace to increase heart rate to 100 - 120 beats per minute (take your pulse for 6 seconds and multiply by 10 to check your heart rate)
3. Gradually increase the time your pulse remains at your target rate by extending your walk as tolerated. Walking should increase your energy after your heart rate returns to normal, without causing fatigue. Do not exercise to a point of causing fatigue; this is not healthy nor recommended.
4. Last 5 minutes, reduce pace to allow your heart rate to return to normal gradually

Do not exercise if you have:

◆ Fever
◆ Nausea or vomiting
◆ Muscle joint pain and swelling
◆ Bleeding from any source
◆ Irregular heart beat
◆ Dizziness or fainting
◆ Chest, arm, or jaw pain
◆ Intravenous chemotherapy administration on same day
◆ Blood drawing on same day—may exercise afterwards, prior exercise may alter counts
◆ Any restrictions placed on exercise activities by a physician

Exercise Precautions During Treatment:

If you are receiving chemotherapy your nurse/physician will alert you if your counts are in a range where exercise is not advised. Ask your nurse when you have your blood drawn if your counts are still in a safe range. Recommendations **not to exercise** are as follows:

1. White blood count less than 3,000 mm^3
2. Absolute granulocyte count less that 2,500 mm^3
3. Hemoglobin/hematocrit less than 10g/dl/25%
4. Platelet count less than 25,000 mm^3

Exercise Tips:

◆ Walk with a partner, if possible
◆ Carry identification with you
◆ Listen to inspirational tapes or your favorite music, if you walk alone
◆ Keep an exercise log or diary to monitor your progress
◆ Exercise the same time of day if possible, to make walking routine
◆ Drink a full glass of water before and after you walk
◆ Walk in a safe area, away from traffic

Exercise During Treatment:

Exercise during treatments—chemotherapy or radiation therapy—has to be self-paced. Only you can determine how much you can tolerate and when you feel up to exercising. Begin at a modest level and gradually increase your length of time. Take into consideration that during treatment there may be periods of decreased performance due to effects of treatment. Do not increase your fatigue by pushing yourself during these times. A walking exercise program can be easily modified to meet your changing needs during treatment; it can be started, suspended, decreased, or accelerated according to your physical energy. You may also want to consider other types of exercise such as biking, swimming or gardening.

Check with your physician to determine if this walking program or any other exercise program is recommended during your recovery. Clinical studies have proven that women who walked four to five times weekly during treatments, for 20 - 45 minutes, had more energy, experienced less depression, nausea, insomnia, gained less weight and required less medication to control side-effects of treatment than women who did not exercise. An exercise program is one thing you can do to promote your own recovery while you are still in treatment.

My Commitment To An Exercise Program:

I will check with my doctor about starting my walking program: (date) _____

I am starting an exercise program: (date) _____

I am going to ask to join me: (person) _____

I am keeping a record of my walking program: (yes/no) _____

I plan to walk: (place) _____

Items I need to start my walking exercise program: (shoes, shorts, shirts, tapes, radio):

_____

Learning The Relaxation Response
The Stress Controller For Better Health

The diagnosis of breast cancer is a very stressful event. After the diagnosis, a continual series of events causes fear and increases stress. Surgical choices, chemotherapy, radiation therapy, dealing with all the changes illness brings—the list of additional stressors that cancer brings goes on and on. A limited amount of stress is helpful and serves as motivation. But the constant stress after a breast cancer diagnosis can become a major contributor to physical and mental fatigue. This fatigue and stress can decrease the quality of your life and slow your recovery.

A fearful or stressed body has the **"fight-or-flight"** response. Our bodies prepare for battle to fight or to run from our attackers. During this time of stress or fear, our heart rate **increases**, our breathing rate increases, our blood pressure increases, our metabolic rate increases and our muscles become tense. Researchers have concluded that chronic arousal of the fight-or-flight state may lead to permanent physiological changes—disease. They have also found that the process can be altered by practicing **relaxation techniques**.

The most well-known researcher of relaxation's effects on the body is Dr. Herbert Benson of Harvard Medical School. Dr. Benson's thirty years of research at Harvard have proven that a person can **consciously reverse** this fight or flight stress by learning the **"relaxation response"** when faced with fears and stressors. (Recommended for additional information: *Relaxation Response* by Dr. Herbert Benson, William Morrow Publishing, 1975; *The Wellness Book: A Comprehensive Guide to Maintaining Health and Treating Stress-Related Illness*, Dr. Herbert Benson, Fireside Publishing, 1993.)

The relaxation response **decreases** the respiratory rate, heart rate, blood pressure, metabolism rate and muscle tension in the body. In other words, the relaxation response is a built-in method of stress control. It can interrupt the fight-or-flight response and the negative effects it produces in your body when you become tense or fearful. It is a method of stress control that you can learn and practice anywhere, anytime, it will not cost you anything and has no negative side effects.

During treatment for breast cancer, you may face many things which cause you to become stressed and fearful creating the fight-or-flight effects in your body. You need a plan to free yourself from the stress of your environment to a state of relaxation. The state of relaxation allows your body to return to the state that is most conducive for recovery. Learning Dr. Benson's techniques for learning to relax, even during stressful or fearful times, can give you the power to remain in control of your physiological response to an event.

How do you learn to relax? It begins with a conscious effort.
- Find a quiet room away from interruptions and sit up straight in a chair
- Place your hands comfortably in your lap and close your eyes
- Select a phrase, prayer or word that gives you a sense of peace, love and safety*
- Take a deep breath very slowly and hold it for a few seconds
- As you breathe out slowly, repeat the phrase or word
- Continue inhaling and exhaling while repeating your phrase for 10 - 20 minutes
- When your mind wanders to another thought, refuse to entertain it and gently bring your thoughts back to your breathing and repetitive phrase
- Open your eyes and gradually re-orient yourself to your surroundings

During relaxation you may feel changes in sensations such as a tingling, a sense of floating, drifting or dropping. This indicates that your body is relaxing, it is returning to a state that allows physical recovery to be optimized. It is suggested that the relaxation response be practiced twice a day or used at anytime you feel stressed or fearful.

Mini Relaxation Responses

Often, there are times when stressful situations arise when we need to gain control, but we cannot leave our environment for a quiet place. Simply decide to concentrate on breathing and repeating your phrase with your eyes open, if necessary. Taking a deep breath increases the oxygen to the brain and clears the thinking. Focusing on a word or phrase* during this time of concentrated breathing interrupts the anxiety situations produce. Doing a mini relaxation response can break the tendency to become over-stressed during an event such as having an IV puncture, going through a diagnostic test, undergoing any new procedure or taking chemotherapy or radiation. Utilize your ability to manage stress, keeping your body in a more relaxed state by practicing the mini relaxation response anytime, anywhere.

*Suggested Words or Phrases:

Select a word or phrase that gives you a sense of peace from this list or choose one of your own not listed.

General:

Love, Peace, Calm, Relax, Healing

Christian:

"Our Father who art in heaven"
"The Lord is my shepherd"
"Lord, Jesus Christ, have mercy on me"

Jewish:

"Sh'ma Yisroel"
"Shalom"
"The Lord is my shepherd"

Visualization Relaxation

Another technique is to replace the repetitive phrase with a mental picture of a scene that brings a sense of peace and safety—a garden, park, seashore, etc. As you breathe slowly, mentally feel and explore the beauty of this favorite place in your mind—smell the fragrances, feel the warmth of the sun, and hear the familiar sounds. Visualization also promotes the relaxation response in your body.

Taking charge of stress and keeping it manageable is a step toward improving mental and physical health. Learning to relax is something you can do to remain in control of your emotions during times of stress, preventing the fight-or-flight response, and creating an environment for your optional recovery.

Personal Plan for Recovery

*"Planning is like a road map. It can show us the way
and head us in the right direction and keep us on course.
Planning means mapping out how to get from here to where we
want to be. Planning is the power tool for achievement,
the magic bridge to our goals and our success."*

~ Wynn Davis

Take the time to plan steps of action in every area of your life for maximum recovery. Inventory your lifestyle and make the adjustments you feel will restore a sense of control.

Support System

Personal: Identify at least two people you can talk to openly.

I can talk to: _____

_____

Information: Identify sources of correct information on breast cancer. Check the resource section of this book.

Physician: _____ Telephone: _____
Physician: _____ Telephone: _____
Nurse: _____ Telephone: _____
Organization: _____ Telephone: _____
Organization: _____ Telephone: _____
Organization: _____ Telephone: _____
Organization: _____ Telephone: _____

Support Groups: Identify your local support groups by calling the American Cancer Society or the National Alliance of Breast Cancer Organizations.

Breast Cancer Patients: _____ Telephone: _____
Mates' Groups: _____ Telephone: _____
Children's Classes: _____ Telephone: _____

Spiritual: Identify people who can help you deal with the spiritual aspects of your illness.

_____ Telephone: _____
_____ Telephone: _____
_____ Telephone: _____

187

Personal Plans

❑ **Fears**: Name your fears and plan steps of action to address them. Complete the Fear Management worksheet on page 159.

❑ **Diet:** Evaluate your diet.
I plan to make the following changes: _____

❑ **Exercise:** Plan a program of exercise to restore and maintain your physical condition.
I plan to: _____

❑ **Personal Appearance:** Make plans to enhance your self-esteem and personal appearance during treatment.
I plan to: _____

❑ **Time Management:** Plan to make lifestyle changes: (Employment, Social, Civic duties)
I plan to start: _____
I plan to stop: _____

❑ **Family Management:** Make changes in your household.
I need to delegate chores for: _____
I need to hire help for: _____
I need to stop doing: _____

❑ **Personal Fulfillment:** Think of things you want to do more of or things you want to begin to do. Think selfishly. You deserve it!
I want to begin to add the following goals, hobbies or pleasurable events to my life.
I plan to: _____
_____
_____

❑ **Reaching Out:** A spirit of gratefulness and an effort on your part to help others is very rewarding. Plan to say "thank you" to those who play an important part in your life and recovery. Plan to give back to others who are in need.
People to write or thank: _____
_____
Things I would like to do to help others: _____
_____
_____

Congratulations! You have just taken steps to plan your psychological and social recovery. Refer to this sheet when in doubt of what you can do to speed your recovery.

My Prayer During Breast Cancer

❧ ❧ ❧ ❧ ❧ ❧ ❧ ❧ ❧

Lord, I have just received the diagnosis of breast cancer.
Still my anxious heart as I seek to understand why.
Teach me to transform my suffering into growth,
my great fear of tomorrow into faith in your presence,
my tears into understanding,
my discouragement into courage,
my anger into forgiveness,
my bitterness into acceptance,
my experience with cancer into my testimony,
my crisis into a platform on which
I can learn to help others.
God grant that one day I can embrace this time
as my friend, and not as my enemy.

~ Judy Kneece, RN, OCN

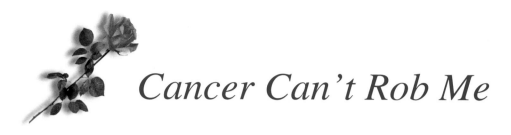

Cancer Can't Rob Me

Today is another new day and I can choose to use it in many ways. I did not choose to have cancer, but I can choose how I am going to respond and what I plan to do with today. Today is mine to make choices. This day can be a new beginning for me, if **I** so choose.

Today can be the day that I decide to exchange those things which weigh my spirit down for a lighter load of faith and trust. I can change my perception of cancer as a "robber" of my health and my future and exchange it into a vehicle to transport me into a life rich in understanding. This understanding will strengthen me and make me valuable to others who will walk the same path after me.

I can choose:
- To see cancer as a "challenge" instead of as a defeat.
- To demystify cancer by learning about my disease rather than cowering in fear of the unknown.
- To give up concentrating on the "things I can't control" and replace them with thoughts of "what I can control."
- To respond with a spirit of "I can" instead of "I can't."
- To ask for help and not try to face the challenge alone.
- To face my fears with a plan for steps of action against them.
- To look for the blessings in the events of today instead of focusing on losses.
- To add to my life the things I have always wanted to do but postponed until the right time. Today is that time.
- To use my spiritual faith as a vehicle to understand why and give me hope.
- To let go of anger, bitterness and resentments which only slow down my recovery.
- To see my cancer experience as a new tool for personal growth,
- To offer my support and share what I'm learning with others who may need my help.

Therefore, I choose for today:
Peace and not anxiety,
Good and not evil,
Love and not hate,
Gain and not loss.

When today becomes tomorrow, this day will be gone forever leaving in its place what I choose today. I, alone, can choose to use today wisely—**Cancer Can't Rob Me Of This Day!**

Judy C. Kneece, RN, OCN